LOSE WEIGHT BY EATING

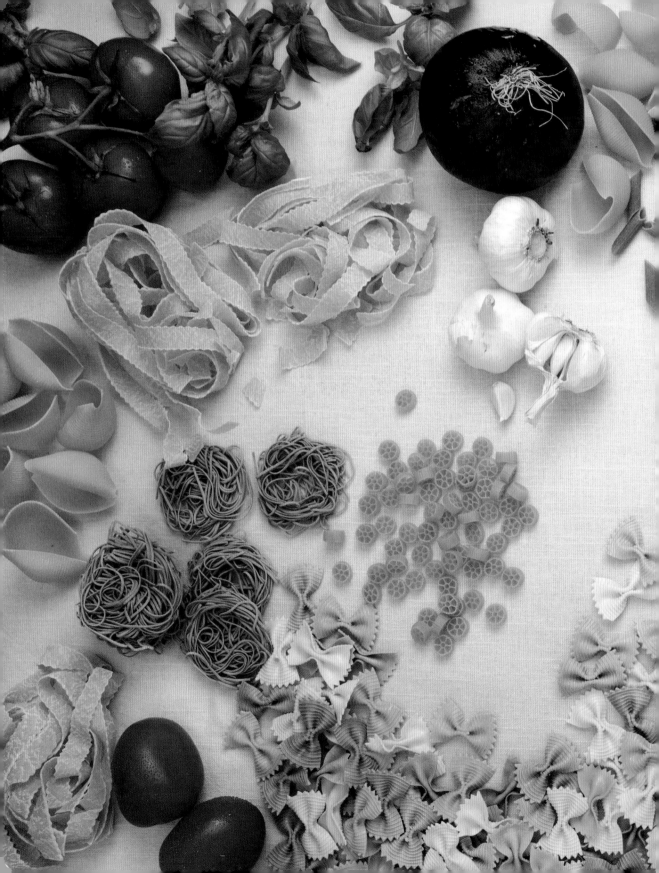

LOSE WEIGHT BY EATING

130 AMAZING CLEAN-EATING RECIPE MAKEOVERS FOR GUILT-FREE COMFORT FOOD

AUDREY JOHNS

wm

WILLIAM MORROW

An Imprint of HarperCollins*Publishers*

This book is written as a source of information only. The information contained in this book should by no means be considered a substitute for the advice of a qualified medical professional, who should always be consulted before beginning any new diet, exercise, or other health program.

HarperCollins books may be purchased for educational, business, or sales promotional use. For information please e-mail the Special Markets Department at SPsales@harpercollins.com.

FIRST EDITION

Designed by Diahann Sturge

Library of Congress Cataloging-in-Publication Data has been applied for.

ISBN 978-0-06-237869-9

16 17 18 19 20   OV/RRD   10 9 8 7 6 5 4 3 2 1

For the amazing women who inspire me:

Mom—You taught me that life was what I made of it and that my dreams could become reality if I had the gumption and drive to make them happen.

Sophia—I hope many of these recipes are the ones you'll ask for during trips home from college. Thank you for helping me shop for, cook, and taste these recipes and for inspiring me to be the kind of mom you can be proud of every day.

CONTENTS

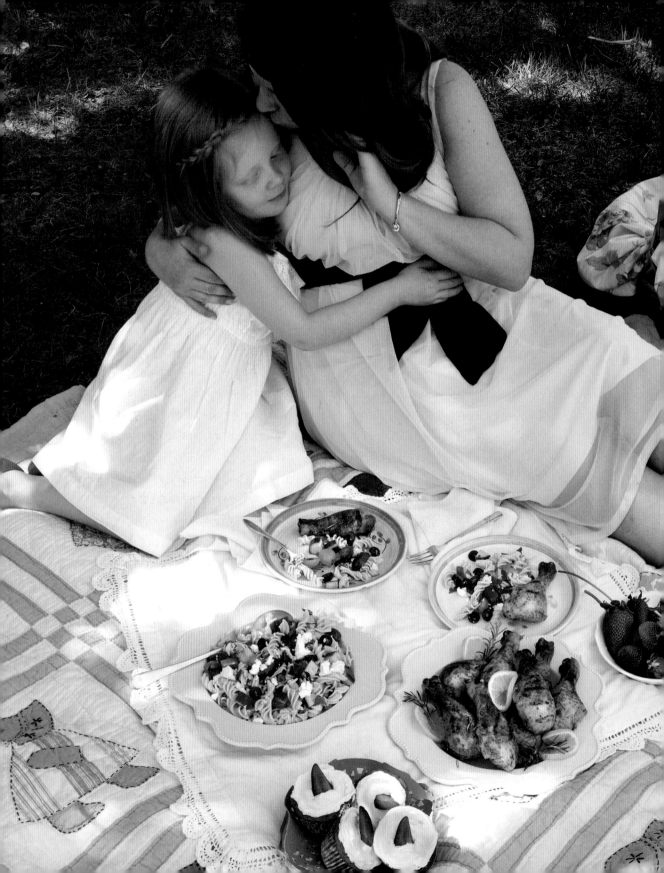

Introduction

The weight-loss industry is a multimillion-dollar business. Every company boasts a weight-loss product that costs a small fortune and fails to leave you with lasting results. What it all really comes down to is marketing. I use the beer analogy often when I try to get through to people who can't cut through the marketing BS; I ask them, "Do you really think when you open a cold can of beer a frozen train will show up at your house?" You don't, that's silly . . . but chances are you've bought into less outrageous diet claims. And that's all they are—claims.

Don't feel bad. I bought into marketing hype for years, but when I finally saw it for what it was and stopped blindly believing what big food companies told me, I lost weight and kept it off for the first time in my life. Before this revelation, I was always the biggest girl in the room, the girl who was always told, "But you have such a pretty face." After trying every major diet out there (and some scary minor ones, too) without any lasting results, I was left heavier than ever, more broke than ever, and depressed. I felt awful and I was nearing the three-hundred-pound mark. Something had to change—but what do you do when you're penny-pinching? The answer was so simple I couldn't believe I had missed it for so many years: just go back to nature and let nature do all the work.

I was eating under 1,000 calories a day of frozen "diet" meals and diet sodas, and all along I was gaining weight. My signature dish was anything that came out of a box and could be made fast—convenience was more important to me than nutrition. No veggies, no wholesome food, all because I thought nutritious food was boring, expensive, and difficult to make. I had been brought up on Shake 'N Bake, boxed side dishes, drive-thru takeout, and quick microwaved meals—and I realized I was bringing my daughter up on them, too.

I started by giving up my first love, the zero-calorie diet soda, and when I lost ten pounds that first week without any other modifications to my diet, I knew I was onto something. The next week I stopped consuming all artificial sweeteners and five pounds flew off, and the following week I dropped another eight pounds by removing preservatives from my diet. I kept it up, and after a short eleven months I had lost 150 pounds. I had gone from a size 24 to a size 4, I felt and looked amazing, and best of all my grocery (and medical) bills had dropped substantially. I hadn't just proved that eating all natural could help you lose weight—I'd proved it was inexpensive as well.

Unfortunately my cravings never stopped, and by month two all I wanted was a burger and fries, some mac and cheese, and my favorite, cookies! I had to find ways to eat what I wanted without reversing all the hard work I'd done. By slightly changing my favorite meals and allowing myself a very lax kitchen learning curve, I found ways to eat the naughty, delicious food I was craving, all while losing pounds and later maintaining my new healthy weight. I cut calories by adding in vegetables and swapping high-calorie ingredients like butter and sugar for all-natural applesauce and mashed fruits. I took mac and cheese from 800 calories per serving to 300 by cutting down on the butter, choosing sharp cheese for extra flavor, and substituting metabolism-boosting almond milk for heavy cream.

I was so excited I wanted to shout my weight-loss breakthrough from the rooftops, so I started my blog, *Lose Weight by Eating,* and posted recipes to share the knowledge with any readers who stumbled across it. In the past I spent a fortune in failed attempts to lose weight. Now that I had found the answer I wanted to share what I'd learned free of charge to the masses, and it paid off for all involved. Women and men who had struggled for years with weight and illness changed their diets, and by doing so they changed their lives for the better. Women whose signature dish was cereal in milk were finally learning to cook, starting with easy yet impressive meals like my Whole Roasted Chicken with Potatoes and Onions (page 200). They told me their boyfriends were so impressed that they finally saw them as wife material. One gal in particular learned to cook from my recipes, got married, bought a small ranch, and now raises her own chickens and writes a popular food column for a local newspaper. Three years ago she couldn't cook, and today she's a food journalist!

That's what I love most about cooking—you don't need to go to school to learn how to cook! Julia Child could barely boil an egg when she was in her late thirties, and look what happened to her. Just a little kitchen confidence and you can change your life, your body, and your health.

The recipes on my blog and the *Lose Weight by Eating* plan have helped thousands of people. A woman in her seventies who thought weight loss was impossible lost almost 170 pounds. A sixteen-year-old started cooking my recipes for her family, resulting in a family-wide hundred-pound weight loss, a new healthy lifestyle, and some seriously impressive kitchen confidence for a high schooler. A man with a knee injury who could no longer hit the gym found solace and weight loss in his kitchen. All these amazing people have inspired me ten times more than I ever inspired them. Their weight-loss success stories have helped me prove that if you can wield a spatula, you can lose weight—it all comes down to what you eat.

So why trust me that healthy food can be delicious? James Beard Award–winning chef Marcus Samuelsson picked me out of thirty-six people to be on his team of four on Season 2 of ABC's *The Taste*. And you'd trust him to know good food, right? Of the other judges, Nigella Lawson told me that the world needs my food, Anthony Bourdain said I cook pasta as well as any chef, and even hotheaded Ludo Lefebvre claimed that my Garlic Roasted Potatoes (page 226) were some of the best potatoes he'd ever had. If this stay-at-home mom living in a rural town in California can learn to cook well, lose weight, and make it into a national cooking competition all in three years, you certainly can, too.

This book is all about making the naughty *nice*. The foods you crave may make you gain weight, but you can give them a delicious makeover with some simple (and inexpensive) "Smart Swaps" so you *can* eat them every day. Want to lose weight eating pizza, cookies, meat loaf, and nachos? Well then, *Lose Weight by Eating* is for you. Life is too short to eat boring, bland "diet" food . . . so let's get cooking. What do you have to lose but the weight?!

· *Chapter 1* ·

Lose Weight by Eating

I want you to forget all the weight-loss "rules" you've learned over the years and read this chapter with a fresh, open mind. We demonize food and calories, but we can't live without them. We look for zero-calorie snacks in the hope that they'll fill us up (they never do) but don't realize we're missing an opportunity to feed our bodies fat-burning fuel. Food is not the problem—food-*like* products are. They are the reason millions of people can't lose weight or maintain the figure they want.

The delicious recipes in this book will give your body the fuel it needs to lose weight, and with added metabolism-boosting ingredients, they'll actually do the weight-loss work for you! I've given the recipes a nip and tuck to cut calories and fat. It's hard to imagine that meat loaf could actually help you lose weight, but mine does! By swapping the beef for turkey, adding some hidden veggies, and topping it with some homemade all-natural red wine barbecue sauce, you'll be feeding your cravings and burning extra fat. When testing recipes for this book, I had one main objective: make them just as delicious as their full-fat, high-calorie versions. If they weren't, then they got cut from the book. I tried to make skinny onion rings five times, then finally gave up and cut the recipe. My promise to you: If the recipe was not totally amazing, I didn't add it, period.

Of course eating an entire tray of skinny brownies isn't going to help you lose weight, no matter how many calories I cut from the recipe, so be sure to look at serving sizes and stay within them. If you want seconds or thirds, go for veggies or a salad—you can have unlimited raw and steamed veggies and salads with all-natural dressings, so go nuts and get your veggies in! Vegetables are an important part of your diet. Our long-ago ancestors didn't have grocery stores; they ate what they could find or could grow for themselves. It's important to remember that we need to feed ourselves what we ate when we lived more natural lives—just like our pets, we are animals, too. You wouldn't feed your dog or cat ice cream or brownies; you feed them what their bodies need. That's where veggies come in. Just as pain receptors tell you that fire is burning your hand, we have hunger receptors, and the only way to turn them off for hours is to give them what they truly crave: vegetables. You can sit down and eat a bucket of fried chicken, then two hours later you're mysteriously hungry again. Why is that? Because your body didn't get what it truly craved.

Ideally you want your plate to be 50 percent vegetables, 25 percent lean protein, and 25 percent whole grains. This well-rounded plate will turn off your hunger receptors, increase your metabolism, and keep you full for hours. Don't worry if you're not a veggie fanatic; I hid veggies in most of these recipes, so you may not notice you're eating them, but your hunger receptors will. (But you can't always hide your veggies, and when they're front and center, they'd better be delicious! Try my Guide to the Perfect Salad on page 18 and create some crunchy new favorites for yourself.)

Four Goals to Reach For

The *Lose Weight by Eating* plan is very easy to follow because there are no rules, only goals. Set rules for yourself and all you'll want to do is break them. Set goals for yourself and you'll strive to meet, even beat them, and if you mess up, don't worry—tomorrow is a new day and a fresh start! Here are the four goals you'll be reaching for:

- Skip the processed food and drinks and go all natural.
- Start planning your meals and log everything you eat and drink.
- Get your body moving.
- Drink a gallon of water a day.

Skip the Processed Food and Drinks and Go All Natural

So, what's "all natural"? All-natural food is made with raw, unprocessed ingredients. For example, all-natural peanut butter contains only one ingredient: peanuts. But peanut butter made from peanuts, oil, sugar, salt, and preservatives is processed, not all natural. Processed foods tend to be lower in nutrients and higher in calories, but all-natural peanut butter is full of protein, omega-3 fatty acids, zinc, and iron (among many other nutrients) to give you shiny hair, strong nails, and improved skin tone (think "youthful glow"). All-natural food has many benefits, but weight loss, better health, and looking younger are my personal favorites.

What's wrong with processed food? It's filled with preservatives, chemical-derived thickening agents, and fake sugars, all of which have been proven to cause weight gain. So if you think your meal of a frozen "diet" dinner, zero-calorie soda, and 100-calorie "sugar-free" frozen treat is helping you lose weight, you're just being fooled. The preservatives in the dinner are storing fat in your body, the diet soda is rotting your teeth and causing weight gain, and the artificial colors and sweeteners in the frozen treat will leave you craving more sweets and carbs. On the other hand, my Veggie-Packed Lasagna (page 156) with Homemade Blueberry Orange Soda (page 260) and a scoop of Pineapple Mango Ginger Sorbet (page 252) will leave you satisfied, with your metabolism roaring for hours and your skin glowing. Which would you choose?

Processed food has literally taken over our grocery stores, pushing all the real food to the perimeters. So I use this to my benefit and shop only the perimeters of the store. The produce department is my first stop, for organic fruits and veggies; then I hit up the butcher counter for some organic lean protein; and finally I visit the bakery for some store-baked bread. I also love to shop like my great-grandmother did. I go to the local, organic, GMO-free farmers' collective for my produce and grains, the local bakery that makes hands down the best bread ever, and my organic butcher, which moved in next to my favorite grocery store, Trader Joe's, where I shop for pantry staples like Dijon mustard and tomato paste. Just remember, wherever you choose to shop, look for organic and GMO-free food whenever possible.

If I ever call for an ingredient you're unsure of and you're lucky enough to have a local Trader Joe's, ask a staff member for that ingredient, as I shopped almost exclusively at TJ's for the recipes in this book.

I've found that I save more than $200 per month by shopping for all-natural food, and it's mainly because I'm no longer buying boxes of premade snacks or expensive frozen dinners and drinking water instead of buying sodas. The cost savings were enough to convince me at first, but I quickly loved that I knew what was in everything I was eating instead of blindly trusting the big food companies. I felt good about feeding my six-year-old daughter food that would nourish her body instead of just filling up her belly. Food is so much more than just calories and flavor; it's fuel for your body, and feeding yourself processed food is like putting diesel in your unleaded-gas-only car.

Start Planning Your Meals and Log Everything You Eat and Drink

No one likes homework, but I promise this homework will save you money, time, calories, and your sanity! I've included meal-planning menus on pages 274–279 and at loseweightbyeating.com to make your homework less cumbersome and more enjoyable.

Meal planning is a great way to save money and stay on track. Place the meal planner on your fridge or in your day planner so that you feel in control all week. Best of all, you're less likely to splurge and go off plan when you know you have an amazing dinner lined up in just a few hours. While filling out the meal planner, choose recipes that you can make extras of and freeze in individual containers for homemade frozen lunches and dinners, make extra protein and use it up all week in salads and sandwiches, and if you buy a big bunch of cilantro, look for other recipes in the book that use it so that you don't let it go to waste. A little research and time on Sunday or Monday will save you hours later in the week.

I always encourage people to plan for their cravings, not to fight them! If you have a daily three P.M. carbohydrate craving, be sure to have enough carbs at lunch. A sandwich or leftover Skinny Chicken Alfredo (page 146) is great to curb afternoon carbohydrate cravings. Do you crave sweets at 10:30 A.M. every day (like I do)? Then make some of the Strawberry Scones with Lime Glaze (page 60) for next week's breakfasts, or enjoy some Homemade Pumpkin Spice Granola (page 34) in the morning. Planning for these cravings will help you feel more satisfied; the more satisfied you feel, the longer you'll want to stick with it and the more weight you will lose. Not quite sure what your cravings are? Then it's time to find out—start logging your food now! Go ahead and start enjoying the healthy meals in this book, writing down everything you eat. In four to six weeks, take a look at your food logs and highlight any consistencies. This will show you all your cravings, even the ones you're trying to hide from yourself.

So why do you need to log your food if you have a meal planner? Because life never goes as planned. On pages 16–17, I've included a log for you to photocopy and fill out each week. (You can also download and print a copy from loseweightbyeating.com.) Carry your log with you in your purse or day planner or stick it on your fridge. Log all your food, drinks, and water. Keep these logs in a binder, and if you hit a plateau, go back and look at your progress. Check for inconsistencies. Analyze the weeks you did exceptionally well and mimic them.

Again, I know this may feel like homework, but this homework will set you up for success for the rest of your life. After about six months of logging your food, you'll be able to look at raw foods at the store and know the apples are 70 calories each, the cucumbers 50 calories each, and the eggs 75 calories each. You'll eventually have memorized 75 percent of the ingredients you typically purchase, and after some time (about nine months) you'll be able to stop logging your food altogether, returning to your food logs only to overcome plateaus or refresh your motivation. So study up, because your life is the test and you're already halfway through it, babe.

Get Your Body Moving

Weight loss is 70 percent diet and 30 percent exercise, so you don't need to be a marathon runner or a Zumba instructor to get the figure you've always wanted. I have many clients who are disabled or recovering from injuries and can't hit the gym in a traditional way, but they still lose weight and keep it off. How do they do it? They find ways to move their bodies more each day, from kicking butt at physical therapy to dancing in their living rooms during commercial breaks, to parking farther away for a few extra steps, to the always popular taking the stairs over the elevator.

Set a reasonable exercise goal each week. Start with increasing your exercise time by one hour this week. If you don't exercise at all, your goal is to work out for one hour this week. If you exercise four hours per week, then strive for five this week. Increase your time by one hour each month until you're working out seven hours per week. Find something you love to do and turn it into an exercise. Do you love to shop? Then walk around the mall at a fast pace from end to end. Enjoy the water? Swim laps. Feel like you need your own quiet time? Pop in a yoga video. You don't have to have a gym membership to work out—you just need to think outside the box. Exercise will speed up your weight loss while it helps you feel good physically and mentally, so it's time to find some exercise you will enjoy.

People often ask me about my 150-pound weight loss, and one of the questions I'm often asked, shyly, is "What about the extra skin?" My answer is exercise, babe! You can technically lose the weight without exercising, but if you want to tone up that extra skin, then you've got to get your muscles working! I also recommend you hit up the raw vitamin C, which helps improve the collagen in your skin, increasing its elasticity and helping your body tighten up as you lose the weight. Many of my recipes are packed full of vitamin C, as it also happens to increase your metabolism. Choose citrus-packed recipes like Orange Cream Popsicles (page 254) and oranges, apricots, or berries to snack on.

Drink a Gallon of Water a Day

Water is the single most important ingredient in weight loss! It fills you up, detoxes your body, and naturally raises your metabolism. Many of my clients often find that they're already drinking close to a gallon a day, while others have great difficulty with their water intake. To help all of them consistently meet this daily goal, I've created many popular fruit-infused water recipes (heck, I wrote a book of them!). This is the healthy alternative to the "zero-calorie" packets of chemical flavoring that only hinder your weight loss.

I encourage you to drink water in place of all your other daily drinks, allowing for one cup of coffee per day and two optional skinny cocktails (my Blueberry Mint Vodka Spritzers, page 265, and Watermelon Margaritas, page 270) per week. Diet sodas are known to cause weight gain and fat storage; plus, they ruin your teeth and contribute to other health problems. It's time to move on from that abusive relationship and into a healthy one with water. That goes for most of the fake sugars out there—avoid sports drinks and just about anything that says "sugar-free" or "zero calories" on the label (raw stevia being the exception, and even that should be consumed in moderation, as it can cause carbohydrate and sugar cravings).

I've included a few water recipes, like my Skin-Firming Citrus Boost Water (page 262), to help you drink more water and kick any soda addictions, and here are some of my favorite water-drinking tips to help get you there faster:

- Drink two 8-ounce glasses of water with each meal. That gets you close to a half gallon right there.
- Buy a 24-ounce BPA-free-plastic or glass water bottle and drink a little over five a day (my preferred method), drinking one with each meal and carrying it around all day.
- Set an alarm on your phone to remind you to drink water. This is great if you're busy or forgetful—and that's most of us!
- Tally your water intake in your food journal (see page 14).
- Add fresh or frozen fruit to your water. Frozen fruit is more fun and delicious than ice cubes. I have a friend who keeps a packet of frozen mixed berries on hand to use in place of ice cubes.
- Fizzy water is one of my favorite ways to drink water. I love it when restaurants have club soda on their unlimited fountain soda machines. Sometimes I put my fizzy water in a wineglass at dinner and sip it as I would sip wine. Guilt-free and fun! Add fruit and make your own sodas (see page 260).

The Lose Weight by Eating *SECRET WEAPON* . . .

Don't forget your reset button! We all mess up and have an extra cookie or forget a workout. Every single person does this, even me. You've no doubt heard it and you've probably said it: "I'll start again on Monday." The people who are successful in weight loss don't just give up when they mess up; they hit their reset button. Don't justify blowing the entire day because of one bad decision. Don't say to yourself, "I already blew today, so I might as well go nuts," and certainly don't punish yourself by skipping your next meal. Just hit your reset button and move on.

You *will* mess up—it *will* happen—so how are you going to handle it? Will you power on or will you give up? I implore you to hit that reset button and get over it—no self-guilt, no binge eating. If you can master your reset button, you'll lose the weight, period!

Setting Weight-Loss Goals and Measuring Success

Now let's talk about your expectations. I want to remind you that everyone loses weight at his or her own pace, and you do need to give yourself reasonable weight-loss goals. Expecting to lose ten pounds the first week is not reasonable; sure, it might happen, but what happens when you lose only three pounds? You could become discouraged and give up. While a three-pound loss is great (that's more than 150 pounds in twelve months!), you need to set goals you can reach so you can celebrate a win each week and feel good about yourself. You can always beat those goals, but starting with reasonable, attainable goals is paramount.

I have helped thousands of people lose weight in a healthy, delicious way that's easy to maintain, and while many have lost big numbers in the first four weeks (ten to seventeen pounds), I encourage you to look at the long game, not the short one. Instead of obsessing over weekly weight-loss results, take an average!

To illustrate my point, see the weekly weight-loss calculations from two of my clients:

- Client 1 weight loss per week in pounds: –9, +1, –2, –4, 0, –3, +2, –5 = 20 pounds in 8 weeks (average 2.5 pounds per week)
- Client 2 weight loss per week in pounds: –3, –2, –2.5, –3, –1.5, –2.5, –3.5, –2 = 20 pounds in 8 weeks (average 2.5 pounds per week)

As you can see, both clients landed in the same place once we look at the average. Client 1 rejoiced week one, wanted to give up week two, and was less than happy with week three. This emotional weight-loss roller coaster went on and on until I showed her the eight-week average, which left her thrilled with her progress.

Client 2 was less than impressed and thought something was wrong. Why wasn't she losing weight as quickly as other clients? Instead of focusing on her good fortune of consistent, steady weight loss, she lusted after the big numbers of people like Client 1, never paying attention to the weeks that client gained but fixating only on her big loss weeks. Once I showed her she was losing exactly the same amount, she was thrilled and proud of her hard work.

So before you decide if you're happy with your weight-loss numbers or not, take an eight-week average and stay patient. If you're a woman, you most likely have one week per month when you hold on to extra water weight. Once you see the patterns and averages, you'll have a better grasp of your success, and you'll begin to know your body better, too. Use the following table to log your weight loss. Tape it on the wall above your scale and fill it in each week.

If you're anti-scale, find a way to measure success in weight loss, not for vanity but so you know what you're doing is working. You can use a tape measure and log your inches, try on the same pair of too-tight skinny jeans and measure the distance until they button, or have your BMI checked weekly (WebMD has a great free BMI calculator)—just find a way to measure that you're comfortable with. If you find that it isn't working at any time, reread this chapter and go through your food logs—I call it "going back to basics" and do it often myself. Most likely you'll find an area where you can improve or an ingredient you didn't realize was affecting your weight loss in a negative manner.

WEIGHT LOSS LOG

Every little bit adds up. Don't be discouraged by a low weight-loss week—next week will be better!

A 2.5-pound weight loss per week equals 130 pounds in a year. Remember, slow and steady wins the race.

Date	Number of pounds lost or gained

Total # of pounds lost: _____ ÷ 8 = _____ (total eight-week average)

A Little Housekeeping Before We Get Started

Food Quality

Organic and GMO-free foods are always preferred—they'll have fewer pesticides, bringing the ingredients closer to nature. Some (but not all) organic or GMO-free items will be much more expensive, and I understand that not everyone can afford a 100 percent organic, GMO-free diet, so you'll want to compare the prices. For instance, organic sugar and flour are about one dollar more per bag; that's worth the extra dollar, so get them. I always go organic for fruits and veggies, but if you can't, buy organic only if you eat the outermost part, such as with apples, asparagus, and salad greens. If you discard the peel, as with bananas, avocados, and mangos, it's less harmful to buy conventionally grown produce. But if you can afford it, go all organic. Think about your health care savings later in life. Take care of your body now and it will take care of you later. It's the best investment you can make!

Ingredients

If I call for almond milk and you're allergic, buy coconut milk or 1% milk—just always choose the unsweetened original. Same for 0% Greek yogurt—if you're vegan, get unsweetened vegan yogurt. You can always add sweetness later, plus with unsweetened products you can also make savory dishes like Creamy Mac and Cheese (page 90) and rich salad dressings. Always choosing the most plain or basic ingredient will save you money and stretch your groceries further.

I make a lot of my own ingredients, such as my Homemade Applesauce (page 112) and Skinny Pesto (page 71), but if you buy them, choose unsweetened applesauce, and always read the ingredient label on the pesto to make sure it's made with whole ingredients. If you can pronounce the ingredients, they're probably safe.

My Magic Ingredient

I absolutely adore my olive oil spray! I call for it often in this book, but I want to be very clear—do not buy the cans of cooking spray you find in the oil section! They're full of unpronounceable chemicals, nothing you want to be putting in your body. Instead, invest ten dollars in a Misto sprayer and fill it with your own olive oil. You can find a Misto sprayer at many kitchen and household stores, as well as online and on loseweightbyeating.com. It's a fun little kitchen gadget that reminds me of the pump-it-yourself aerosol-free hairsprays from the early 1990s. You pump the can to create pressure so that you can spray a very fine mist of all-natural olive oil. It's well worth the investment as you'll never again have to buy canned cooking spray—just fill up the Misto with the oil you already buy.

WEEKLY FOOD LOG

	Monday	Tuesday	Wednesday
Water			
Breakfast			
Lunch			
Dinner			
Snacks			
Total Calories			

Thursday	Friday	Saturday	Sunday

GUIDE TO THE PERFECT SALAD

Salads are easy enough to make and we know we should eat them more often, but how do you make one that your family will gobble up and beg for more? There's an equation—trust me. I may not be a math scholar, but I am a salad scholar, so put on your fancy reading glasses and take notes . . . this will be on the test at the end of the semester. The equation is one part homemade dressing, one part crisp greens, one part crunch, and one part healthy fat, plus the optional extra credit of add-ins and protein.

STEP 1: DRESSING

Make your own! The stuff in the store is full of chemicals that can cause fat storage and weight gain. Plus it's really easy and you probably already have the ingredients on hand. Just toss everything into a jar, close the lid, and shake it up—and it tastes even better if you make it up to 24 hours in advance!

STEP 2: GREENS

Get some organic greens, and please skip the boring, nutrition-less iceberg. Pick one or mix two of the greens together. My favorite combo is peppery arugula and metabolism-boosting baby spinach.

STEP 3: CRUNCH

Crunch is very important to a salad. Nuts and crispy fruits and veggies, like apples and bell pepper, add depth. Without crunch you might end up with a mushy, boring salad.

STEP 4: HEALTHY FAT

The word "fat" still has a bit of a negative connotation, but it's fading as people begin to understand the role that healthy fats play in a good diet. And it pulls your entire salad together! I love avocado and cheese—both give the creamy texture you need in a salad.

EXTRA CREDIT: ADD-INS

Pick one to three add-ins to pull your salad together. Frozen corn and dried cranberries are great options because they're available year-round and they keep well.

EXTRA CREDIT: PROTEIN

If you're serving the salad alongside a main course, you can skip this part, but a good protein will help keep you full longer. Yes, you can use nuts for both crunch and protein.

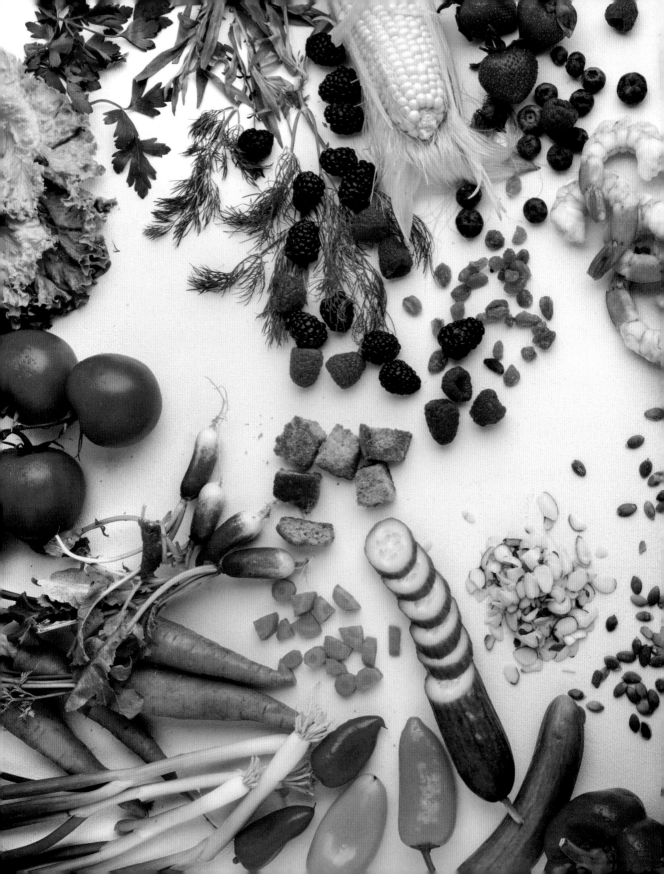

HERE'S THE SALAD SETUP IN REAL-LIFE PRACTICE!

STEP 1: PICK YOUR DRESSING

- Caesar (page 72)
- Blue cheese (page 108)
- Ranch (page 105)
- Citrus vinaigrette (1 tablespoon extra-virgin olive oil, 1 tablespoon apple cider vinegar or champagne vinegar, juice of 1 orange, 1 chopped garlic clove, and salt and pepper to taste)
- Honey mustard (1 teaspoon honey, 1 tablespoon balsamic vinegar, 1 tablespoon extra-virgin olive oil, 1 tablespoon mustard, juice of 1 orange, 1 chopped garlic clove, and salt and pepper to taste)

STEP 2: PICK YOUR GREENS

- Arugula
- Baby spinach
- Romaine
- Field greens

STEP 3: PICK YOUR CRUNCH

- Croutons (page 72)
- Toasted nuts
- Chopped carrots
- Chopped bell peppers
- Chopped apples or pears
- Shredded red cabbage

STEP 4: PICK YOUR FAT

- Avocado
- Cheese
- Nuts
- Hemp, sesame, or sunflower seeds

STEP 5: PICK YOUR ADD-INS

- Frozen corn
- Apple chunks
- Sliced cucumber
- Fresh berries
- Chopped stone fruit
- Chopped green onions
- Raisins or dried cranberries
- Fresh herbs
- Cooked quinoa
- Roasted veggies

STEP 6: PICK YOUR PROTEIN

- Cooked turkey bacon
- Cooked chicken
- Cooked steak
- Cooked shrimp
- Beans
- Cooked tofu

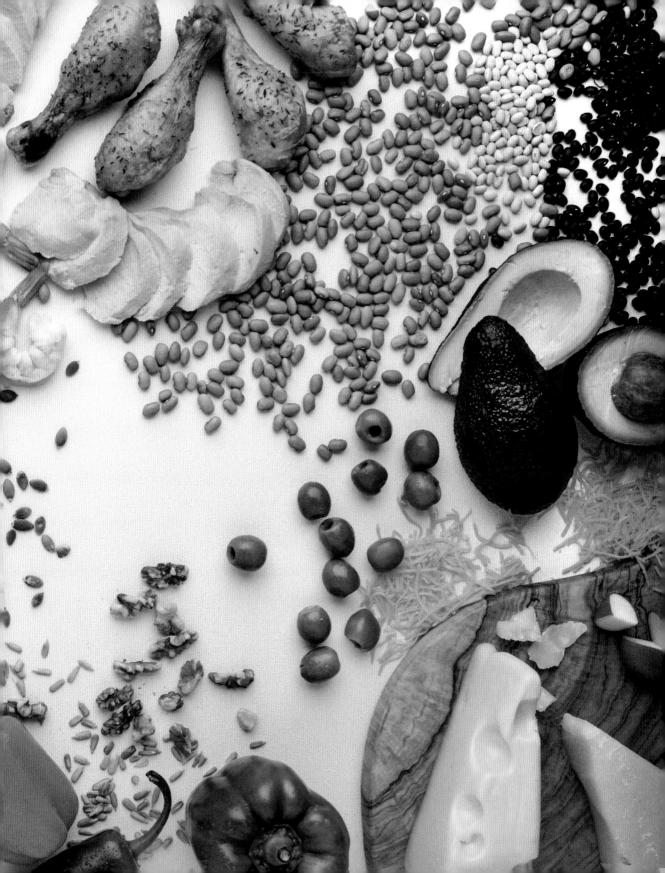

• *Chapter 2* •

Sweet and Hearty Breakfasts

Good morning, beautiful! Let's start your day off right with a filling, healthy breakfast that will set you up for success all day long. Breakfast will get your metabolism roaring early and give your body the fuel it needs to get going. You wouldn't drive your car around all day on empty, then fill up at night before parking it in your garage, would you? Give your body the fuel it needs.

In this chapter, I included all the yummiest, naughtiest breakfast recipes I could think of, made healthy, of course. From my doughnut obsession to my love for food truck breakfast burritos, I created healthy alternatives to satisfy your food cravings while adding fat-burning ingredients to get your metabolism running.

My favorite Smart Swaps for this chapter:

- **Unsweetened almond milk** is a sweet swap that naturally increases metabolism at only 60 calories per cup. I use it in place of milk, buttermilk, and cream.

- **Sharp cheese** has more flavor, so you don't need as much of it. Use it in place of mild cheese and save some calories.

- **Unsweetened Homemade Applesauce** (page 112) used in place of both butter and sugar will cut calories and fat. Apples also naturally boost metabolism.

Old-Fashioned Oatmeal with Topping Bar

Makes 1 serving
Serving size: about ½ cup cooked oatmeal
Per serving: calories 134; fat 3.5 g; fiber 3 g; protein 3.5 g;
carbohydrates 22 g (nutrition information is just for the oatmeal)

Sometimes I think I was put on this earth to convert people who hate oatmeal. I'm madly in love with this metabolism-boosting, ultra-filling superfood! If you're still shaking your head at the idea of eating oatmeal, check out my Giant Breakfast Cookies (page 32). But if you're willing to give oatmeal another try, here's how this oatmeal may be different (and better) from what you're used to.

I use old-fashioned rolled oats. Unlike quick-cooking oats, they're always hearty, never mushy.

I add delicious toppings, boosting flavor while adding health benefits.

I let my family choose their own toppings. It gives them the illusion of control, and kids are always more apt to eat it if they get to choose what's in it . . . spouses, too!

To make it very easy, this recipe feeds just one person. There are four topping categories for each serving, but I kept the sweet toppings optional because I typically don't add them—this oatmeal is sweet enough for me with the almond or coconut milk—but these sweet yet low-calorie add-ins are all natural and pack a punch. Kids love them!

⅓ cup steel-cut or old-fashioned rolled oats
⅔ cup unsweetened almond or coconut milk

1. In a small saucepan (or medium if you're making several servings), combine the oatmeal and milk. Cover and bring to a boil over medium heat. Reduce the heat to low and let the oatmeal bubble away, mixing a couple of times so the oatmeal doesn't burn, until most of the liquid has been absorbed, about 15 minutes.

2. Remove the saucepan from the heat and let it sit, covered and undisturbed, for 10 minutes.

3. Serve the oatmeal with the following toppings, choosing one from each category:

Toppings

Flavor: Vanilla extract; orange, lemon, or lime zest; 1 teaspoon dark chocolate syrup (page 266); almond butter

Crunch: 1 teaspoon chopped almonds, pecans, or walnuts; chopped apple or pear

Fruit: Chopped banana, strawberries, or peaches; dried cranberries or cherries

Sweetness (optional): Maple syrup; Homemade Applesauce (page 112); blended peaches; smashed bananas

For the Busy Cook: I jump in the shower while the oatmeal is cooking. Once I'm out of the shower, I turn off the heat under the oatmeal, do my makeup, and come back to serve it up. You can make this even on your busiest morning; you just have to plan accordingly.

All-Time Favorite Oatmeal Combos

Serving size for each: about ½ cup cooked oatmeal

Growing up, I loved those little packets of quick, flavored oatmeal, but they're packed full of chemicals that negatively affect weight loss. The hearty oatmeal recipes below are free of preservatives and chemical thickeners.

Fruity Oatmeal

Strawberries and Cream Oatmeal

Per serving: calories 249 ; fat 9 g; fiber 8 g; protein 7 g; carbohydrates 54 g

Peaches and Cream Oatmeal

Per serving: calories 264; fat 9 g; fiber 7 g; protein 8 g; carbohydrates 57 g

Blueberries and Cream Oatmeal

Per serving: calories 272; fat 9 g; fiber 7 g; protein 7 g; carbohydrates 57 g

⅓ cup old-fashioned rolled oats

⅔ cup unsweetened almond or coconut milk

2 tablespoons chopped dried strawberries, chopped dried peaches, or dried blueberries

8 white chocolate chips

1. In a small saucepan, combine the oats, milk, and fruit. Cover and bring to a boil over medium heat. Reduce the heat to low and cook, stirring a couple of times to avoid burning, until most of the milk has been absorbed, about 15 minutes. Remove the saucepan from the heat, fold in the white chocolate chips, and let sit, covered and undisturbed, for 10 minutes before serving.

Maple–Brown Sugar Oatmeal

Per serving: calories 162; fat 5.5 g; fiber 5 g; protein 6 g; carbohydrates 51 g

⅓ cup old-fashioned rolled oats

1 tablespoon maple syrup

1 teaspoon brown sugar

1. In a small saucepan, combine the oats and ⅔ cup water. Cover and bring to a boil over medium heat. Reduce the heat to low and cook, stirring a couple of times to avoid burning, until most of the water has been absorbed, about 15 minutes. Remove the saucepan from the heat and let it sit, covered and undisturbed, for 10 minutes. Serve the oatmeal topped with the maple syrup and brown sugar.

Blueberry Pancakes with Blueberry Syrup

Makes 24 pancakes
Serving size: 2 pancakes and 2 tablespoons blueberry syrup
Per serving: calories 130; fat 1 g; fiber 3 g; protein 3 g; carbohydrates 27 g

I personally can't think of a better way to start the day than with a plate of Blueberry Pancakes with Blueberry Syrup. I created a skinny blueberry syrup, lower in calories than regular syrup, and if you already have the blueberries out, you might as well make the two-ingredient special syrup, too, right?

I love a fat-burning breakfast—it's a great way to start the day! Combine the blueberries with applesauce and almond milk and you have a metabolism-boosting breakfast the entire family will love. Store leftovers in a freezer bag, and during the week you can pop the pancakes in a 200°F oven when you wake up. By the time you're done getting ready, the pancakes will be hot.

Pancakes

1¼ cups whole wheat flour
4 teaspoons baking powder
¾ teaspoon kosher salt
1 cup unsweetened almond milk
½ cup Homemade Applesauce (page 112)
2 large eggs
1 teaspoon pure vanilla extract
1 tablespoon pure maple syrup

Blueberry Syrup

3 cups fresh or frozen blueberries
¼ cup pure maple syrup

Olive oil spray
½ cup fresh or frozen blueberries

1. Make the pancake batter: In a large bowl, combine the flour, baking powder, and salt. Set aside.

2. In a medium bowl, whisk the almond milk, applesauce, eggs, vanilla extract, and maple syrup. Pour the wet mixture into the dry and fold until you have a smooth batter. Don't overmix or you'll have tough pancakes. Let the mixture sit for 10 minutes to 1 hour. It will rise and fluff up a little.

3. Meanwhile, make the blueberry syrup: In a medium saucepan, combine the blueberries and maple syrup over medium heat. Cook until the blueberries pop and bleed, stirring occasionally, about 10 minutes. Remove from the heat (if it cools before serving, you can reheat it briefly as you finish the pancakes).

4. Preheat the oven to 200°F.

5. Heat a griddle or large skillet over medium heat and spray it lightly with olive oil spray. Use a ¼-cup measuring cup to pour the batter onto the hot griddle and immediately drop 4 or 5 blueberries on each pancake. When the pancakes start bubbling all over (not just at the edges), gently flip and cook the other sides for 2 minutes, or until lightly browned on the bottom.

6. As the pancakes are done, transfer them to a baking sheet and place them in the oven to keep warm. Repeat to make the rest of the pancakes.

NOTE: Never squish your pancakes with a spatula, and flip them only once. Good pancakes are fluffy because they've been treated with care. Also, expect that the first pancake will end up in the trash! Ladle out just one pancake the first time so that you don't waste batter.

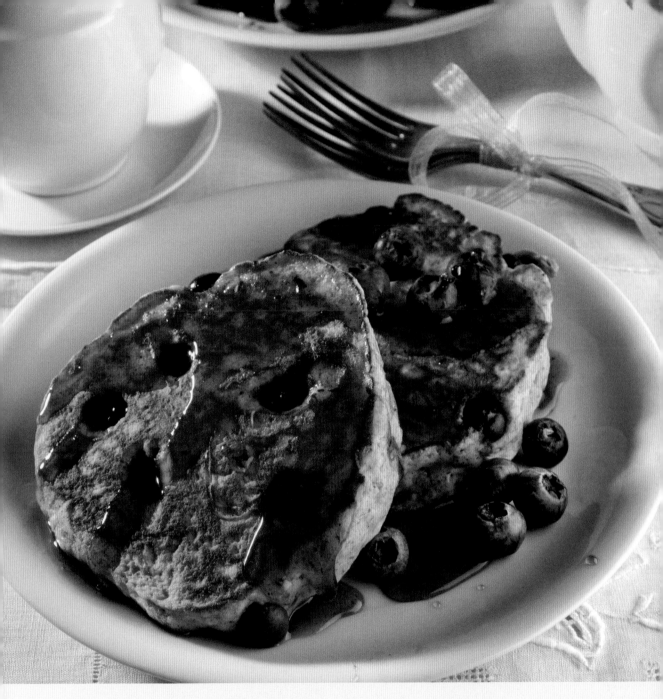

Maple Bacon Pancakes: Substitute crumbled cooked turkey bacon for the blueberries.

Banana Nut Pancakes: Use one large banana, mashed, in place of the applesauce and sprinkle on chopped walnuts in place of the blueberries.

Silver-Dollar Pancakes: Dollop out 2 tablespoons batter for each mini pancake. Dot with blueberries—or not!

Elvis-Inspired Peanut Butter Banana Waffles

Makes 10 waffles
Serving size: 1 waffle
Per serving: calories 188; fat 5 g; fiber 2 g; protein 7 g; carbohydrates 29 g

---

With a child in the house, weekend sleepovers with friends have become a weekly event. Waffles are great for sleepovers—the kids fill up fast and you have leftovers for weekday breakfasts.

I love these peanut butter and banana waffles with a thin layer of peanut butter smeared over the top and a drizzle of maple syrup. They're also great topped with chopped fresh strawberries for a PB&J waffle, and my husband loves these topped with crumbled bacon and maple syrup.

Elvis famously loved peanut butter and banana sandwiches, often with bacon. It was that delicious combo that led to these family-friendly waffles and the Elvis-Inspired Grilled Peanut Butter Banana Panini (page 68). I think the King would approve!

2 bananas
¼ cup all-natural peanut butter
2 large eggs
1 teaspoon pure vanilla extract
1¾ cups unsweetened almond milk
2 cups all-purpose flour
2 tablespoons brown sugar
2 teaspoons baking soda
½ teaspoon kosher salt
Olive oil spray

1. Preheat a waffle maker. Preheat the oven to 200°F.

2. In a medium bowl, use the back of a fork to smash the bananas with the peanut butter. Add the eggs, vanilla, and almond milk and whisk to combine. Set aside.

3. In a large bowl, combine the flour, brown sugar, baking soda, and salt. Fold the wet mixture into the dry mixture and mix until just combined.

4. Spray the waffle maker with olive oil spray. Spoon ⅓ cup batter into the waffle maker and cook until lightly browned, according to the manufacturer's instructions. As the waffles are done, transfer them to a baking sheet and place the sheet in the oven to keep warm. Repeat to make the rest of the waffles, spraying the waffle maker with olive oil spray before adding the batter each time.

5. If you like a crispy waffle, pop it in the toaster for a minute before serving and it will crisp up to perfection.

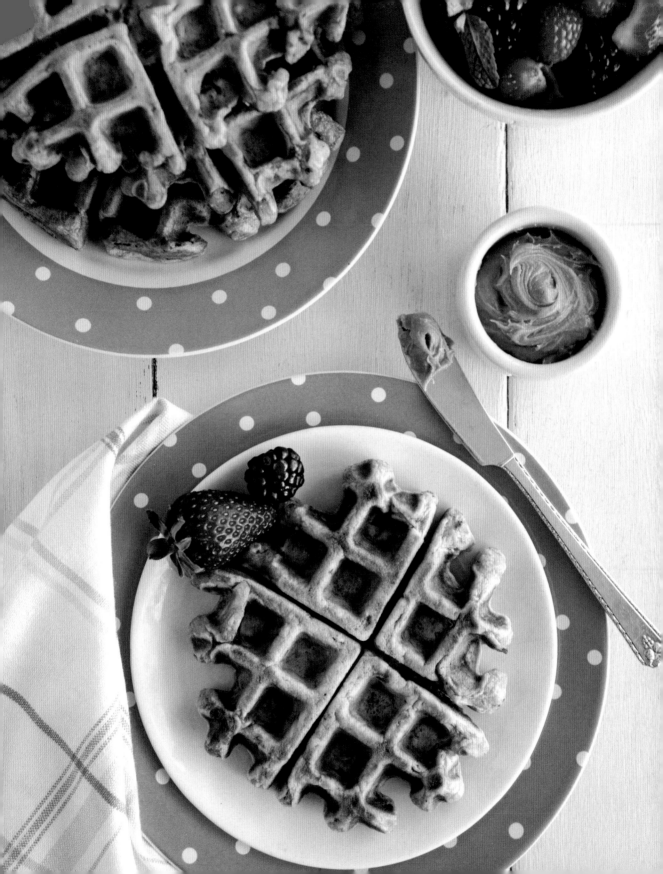

"Jelly Doughnut" French Toast and Strawberry Sauce

Makes 2 servings
Serving size: 2 slices French toast and 2 tablespoons strawberry sauce
Per serving: calories 287; fat 5 g; fiber 7 g; protein 16 g; carbohydrates 40 g

---

French toast sounds so impressive, but between you and me, it's one of the easiest breakfasts you'll ever make! Best of all, you need stale bread to make French toast, so the next time you're about to throw away stale bread, stop yourself and put it in the freezer. You'll have it on hand to make French toast whenever you want.

If you don't have stale bread, just lightly toast the bread in a toaster or oven until it's firmed up a bit, but before it starts to brown. You can also leave the bread out overnight, spread on a baking sheet.

French Toast
Olive oil spray
1 large egg
4 egg whites
1 teaspoon pure vanilla extract
4 slices stale whole wheat bread

Strawberry Sauce
2 teaspoons all-natural strawberry jam
10 strawberries

1 teaspoon powdered sugar, for serving (optional)

1. Make the French toast: Heat a griddle or large skillet over medium-low heat and spray it lightly with olive oil.

2. In a shallow dish or pie tin, whisk the eggs, egg whites, and vanilla until smooth. Dunk the bread into the egg mixture and let it sit for a few seconds to soak. Flip and let the other side soak as well.

3. Place the egg-soaked bread on the hot griddle and cook for 5 minutes on each side, or until the outside is browned and the center is cooked.

4. While the French toast cooks, make the strawberry sauce: In a small food processor or blender, blend the strawberry jam and strawberries until smooth. If you like a chunkier sauce, chop the strawberries and fold together with the jam.

5. To serve, place one slice of French toast on each plate, top with the strawberry sauce, and place another slice of French toast on top. Sprinkle the top lightly with powdered sugar, if desired, and serve with extra strawberry sauce for dunking and drizzling.

Almond-Crusted French Toast: Use ½ teaspoon pure almond extract in place of the vanilla extract. Substitute toasted slivered almonds for the strawberry sauce.

Eggnog French Toast: Add ¼ cup low-fat eggnog to the egg mixture and omit the vanilla extract.

Bellini French Toast: Add ⅛ cup champagne or sparkling wine to the egg mixture and omit the vanilla extract. For the topping, in a small saucepan, combine ½ cup champagne and 1 thinly sliced peeled peach and bring to a boil. Reduce the heat to low and simmer for 20 minutes, stirring often, until you have a smooth sauce and softened peaches. Pour the Bellini sauce over the French toast, spoon on some of the peach slices, and serve.

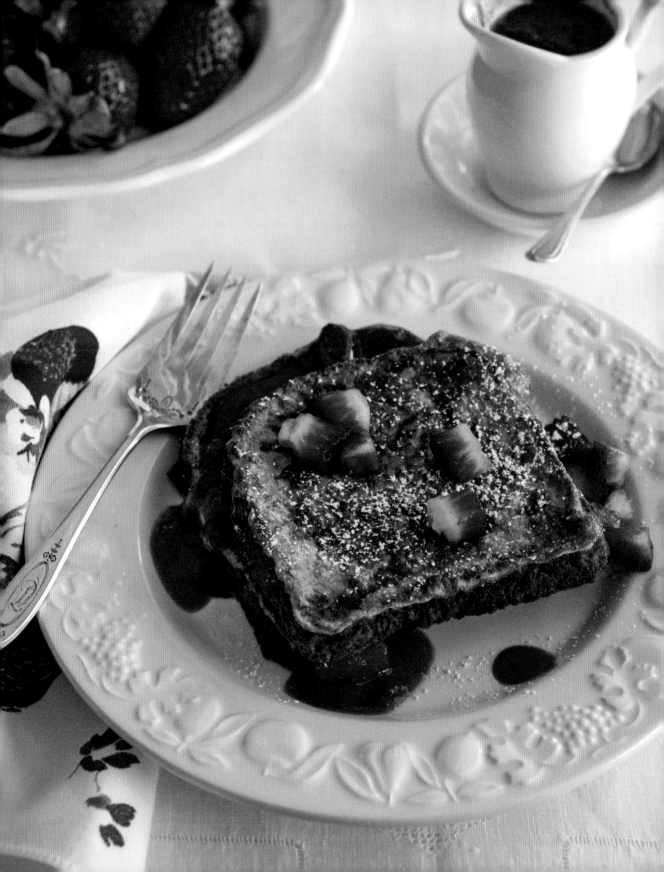

Giant Breakfast Cookies

Makes 15 *big* cookies
Serving size: 1 cookie
Per serving: calories 137; fat 3.5 g; fiber 2 g; protein 3 g; carbohydrates 24 g

---

I was originally going to make breakfast bars with this recipe, but I found that dolloping cookie dough onto a sheet was easier than making bars. Plus, I feel that a cookie looks and tastes more appealing than a breakfast bar a-n-y t-i-m-e! These are basically a bowl of oatmeal baked into cookies, so if you don't like oatmeal, try these instead!

The idea is that you make the cookies at night or on the weekend and then have breakfast ready to grab on the run. You can wrap each one individually in plastic wrap or place the batch in a freezer bag or plastic container. You can store them in the fridge for 1 week or your freezer for up to 3 months.

¾ cup all-purpose flour
½ teaspoon baking soda
Zest of 1 orange
2 tablespoons unsalted butter,
    at room temperature
½ cup packed brown sugar
1 large egg
1 teaspoon pure vanilla extract
½ cup Homemade Applesauce (page 112)
2 cups old-fashioned rolled oats
½ cup dried cranberries
¼ cup sliced almonds

1. In a small bowl, combine the flour, baking soda, and orange zest.

2. In a large bowl or the bowl of a stand mixer fitted with the paddle attachment, whip the butter and sugar until fluffy and pale. Mix in the egg, then the vanilla, applesauce, and ⅓ cup water.

3. Add the dry mixture to the wet mixture and whisk until just combined. Mix in the oats, cranberries, and almonds until just combined. Don't overmix or you'll have tough cookies.

4. Cover the dough with plastic wrap and refrigerate it for at least 15 minutes or overnight to firm it up.

5. Preheat the oven to 350°F. Line two baking sheets with parchment paper.

6. Use an ice cream scoop to place tennis-ball-size dollops of cookie dough on the lined baking sheets, leaving 1½ inches between the cookies to allow for a little spreading. Bake for 15 to 18 minutes, or until golden brown.

7. Transfer the cookies to a wire rack to cool. If you don't have a wire rack, gently lift the parchment paper topped with the cookies and place on a countertop to cool.

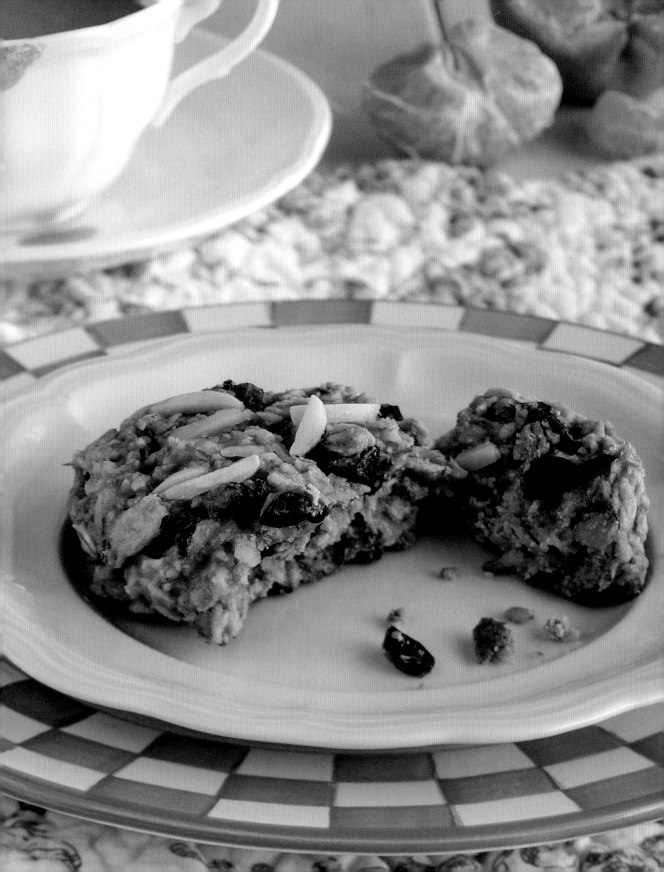

Homemade Pumpkin Spice Granola

Makes 18 servings
Serving size: about ⅓ cup
Per serving: calories 157; fat 9.5 g; fiber 3 g; protein 6 g; carbohydrates 14 g

For this granola recipe I cut out most of the sugar and added ingredients that will give us a beautiful, healthy glow. I recommend that you shop at your local health food store for this recipe; get these ingredients from the bulk section and you can buy only what you need—and save money. If you can find only toasted seeds, they'll do in a pinch, but make sure they're not salted.

This granola goes great over yogurt and as a crunchy snack dry out of a bowl. But I believe it's best served as cereal with almond milk, with Saturday morning cartoons, of course.

1½ cups old-fashioned rolled oats
1½ cups raw pumpkin seeds (pepitas)
1 cup raw sunflower seeds
½ cup slivered almonds
1 (15-ounce) can organic pumpkin puree
¼ cup pure maple syrup
1 teaspoon pure vanilla extract
2 teaspoons pumpkin pie spice
⅓ cup golden raisins

1. Preheat the oven to 350°F.

2. In a 9 x 13-inch pan, combine all the ingredients except the raisins. Mix with a wooden spoon, spread the mixture evenly in the pan, and flatten the top with the back of the spoon.

3. Bake for 30 minutes, then scrape the granola off the bottom of the pan, breaking it into small chunks.

4. Bake for 50 to 60 minutes, stirring and scraping the bottom of the pan every 20 minutes to keep the granola from burning, until the granola is browned and slightly crunchy.

5. Add the raisins and mix the granola. Let it cool in the pan for 3 hours. It will get crunchier as it cools.

6. Store in an airtight container for up to 3 weeks.

NOTE: If you don't have pumpkin pie spice, combine 1 teaspoon ground cinnamon, ½ teaspoon ground ginger, and ½ teaspoon ground nutmeg.

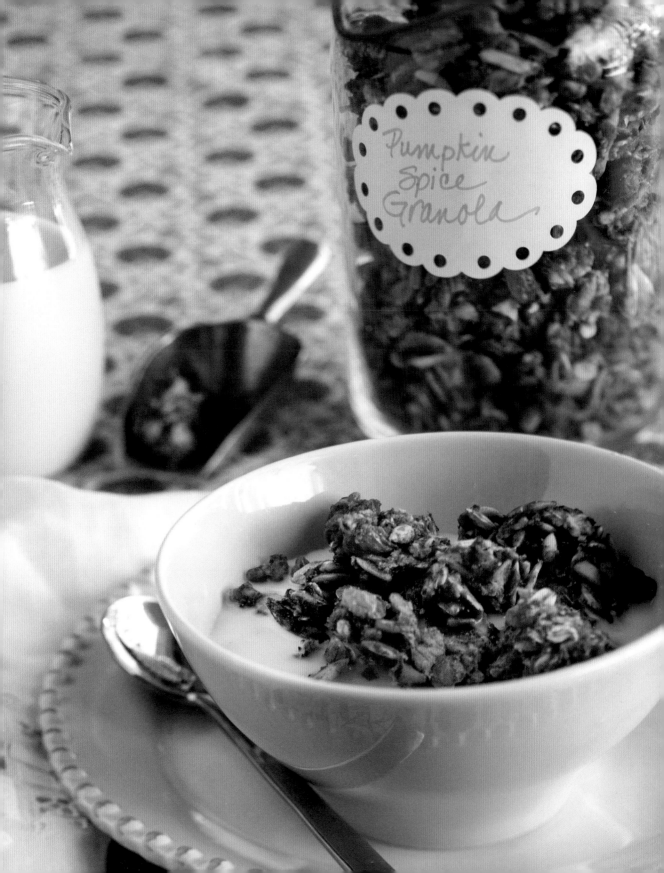

Vegetarian Breakfast Sandwich

Makes 4 sandwiches
Serving size: 1 sandwich
Per serving: calories 367; fat 19 g; fiber 5 g; protein 19 g; carbohydrates 33 g

Eating lots of vegetables is a great way to keep full and satisfied when you're trying to lose weight. With lunch and dinner you can easily add a side salad to increase your vegetable consumption, but a breakfast side salad has yet to become a thing. So I created this yummy sandwich, which is so filling that you won't even miss the meat!

This doesn't have to be a vegetarian meal; see the Note below for some meaty add-ins. It's a delicious way to enjoy a big meal with a lot of healthy ingredients to keep you full and happy for hours.

Olive oil spray
4 large eggs
2 teaspoons garlic salt
1 teaspoon freshly ground black pepper
3 green onions, chopped
4 tablespoons Salsa Ranch Dip (page 105)
8 slices whole wheat bread
  (I like whole wheat sourdough)
¾ cup shredded sharp cheddar cheese
1 avocado, pitted, peeled, and sliced
1 tomato, sliced
1 cup arugula

1. Heat a large skillet over medium heat and spray it lightly with olive oil.

2. In a medium bowl, whisk together the eggs, garlic salt, pepper, and 2 tablespoons water. Pour the mixture into the hot skillet and cook, undisturbed, until the edges start to firm up.

3. Sprinkle the entire pan of eggs with the green onions and use a spatula to cut the eggs into four portions. Fold the edges of the eggs over until the portions are the size of a slice of bread. Cook for another minute, flip, and cook for 2 to 3 minutes more, or until the eggs are done to your liking.

4. While the eggs finish cooking, assemble the sandwiches: Smear 1 tablespoon of the salsa dip on each of 4 slices of the bread and top each with 1 tablespoon shredded cheese. Top the cheese with avocado, tomato, and a second tablespoon of the cheese (you're layering so the cheese holds it all together). Add a handful of arugula (it will wilt and reduce in size when cooked), one portion of cooked egg, and a final tablespoon of the cheese. Top each stack with a second slice of bread.

5. Heat the same pan over medium heat and spray it with olive oil. Add the sandwiches (working in batches as needed), cover the pan, and cook for 5 minutes on each side. When the cheese oozes and the bread is crispy and golden, the sandwiches are ready. Transfer them to a plate, slice them in half, and serve.

NOTE: For a meaty kick, add sliced ham, turkey bacon, or turkey sausage patties.

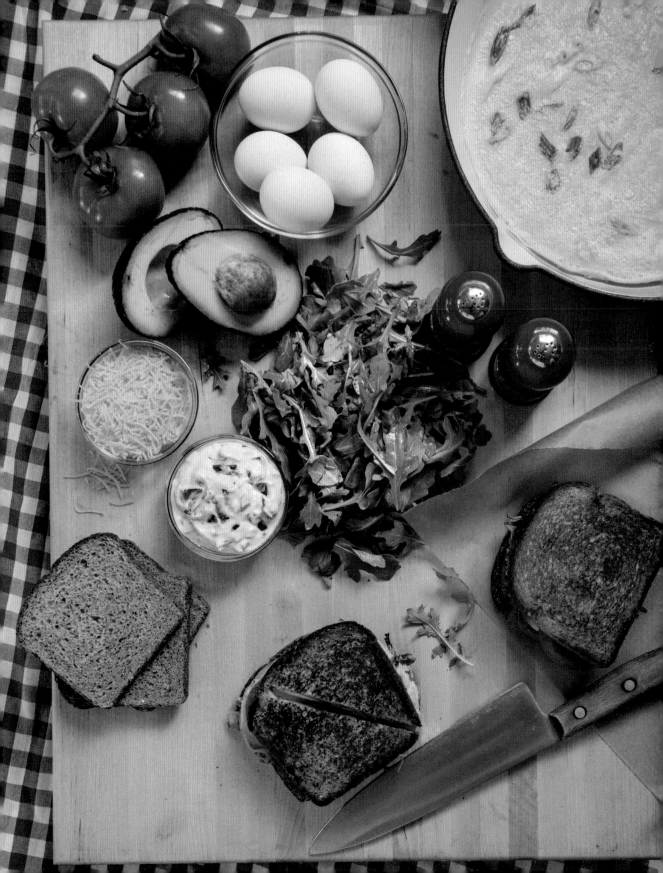

Breakfast Burritos

Makes 4 burritos
Serving size: 1 burrito
Per serving: calories 366; fat 12 g; fiber 5 g; protein 22 g; carbohydrates 43 g

These are easy and delicious, and best of all you can make a double batch on the weekend, assemble the burritos, and freeze them. Then during the week they're just as convenient as burritos you might find in the freezer section of a grocery store—but you'll know exactly what went into them!

I packed these full of veggies to help you fill up with a big breakfast with fewer calories. Hidden veggies are a staple of the Lose Weight by Eating plan; veggies naturally help detox your body while filling you up, turning off your hunger sensors, and increasing your metabolism. Along with the veggies I added cilantro, which is very flavorful and detoxes you naturally, attracting metals in your body and carrying them out. If you're not a fan of cilantro, use chopped fresh parsley, which acts like a loofah for your insides.

Olive oil spray
1 large russet potato, unpeeled,
    cut into ¾-inch cubes
1 onion, chopped
½ red bell pepper, chopped
1 clove garlic, chopped
4 chicken or turkey breakfast sausage links
2 tablespoons chopped fresh cilantro
Kosher salt and freshly ground
    black pepper
2 large eggs
4 egg whites
4 whole wheat tortillas
½ cup shredded Monterey Jack, cheddar,
    or cotija cheese
Hot sauce or salsa (optional)

1. Heat a large skillet over medium-high heat. Spray it lightly with olive oil, add the potato, and cover. Sauté the potato until almost cooked, about 10 minutes, then add the onion, bell pepper, garlic, and sausage. Lower the heat to medium, cover, and cook for 15 minutes, stirring often to avoid burning, until the sausage links are browned and cooked through.

2. Remove the sausage links from the pan and slice them into bite-size chunks. Return them to the pan and brown on all sides, about 5 minutes.

3. Transfer the vegetable-and-sausage mixture to a bowl. Add the cilantro and salt and black pepper to taste, and set aside.

4. Return the skillet to the stovetop over medium heat and lightly spray it with olive oil.

5. In a medium bowl, whisk the eggs, egg whites, and 1 teaspoon water, then add the egg mixture to the hot skillet. Use a wooden spoon to push and scrape the eggs until you have runny scrambled eggs, about 5 minutes. Add the vegetable-and-sausage mixture to the eggs and mix until the eggs are cooked through, about 2 minutes.

6. Spoon ⅓ cup of the scrambled eggs onto each tortilla. Top each with 2 tablespoons cheese and some hot sauce or salsa, if using. Roll up the burritos and serve.

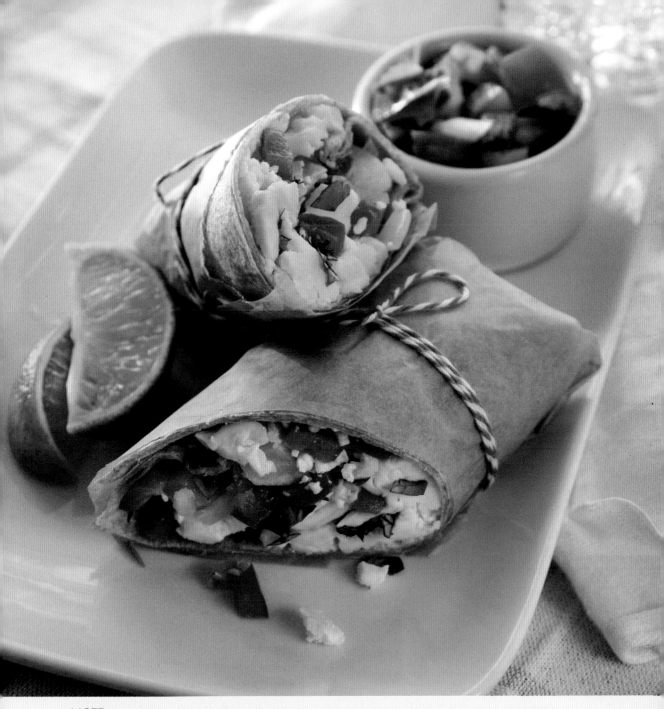

NOTE: If you're freezing the burritos, roll each one in a sheet of aluminum foil, wrap in plastic wrap, and place in the freezer. To reheat, remove just the plastic wrap and bake at 350°F for 15 minutes, or unwrap both the plastic wrap and the foil and microwave for 2 to 4 minutes.

For vegetarian breakfast burritos: Subsititute ½ cup chopped mushrooms for the sausage and use a whole bell pepper. Skip step 2.

Chili Cheese Omelet

Makes 2 omelets
Serving size: 1 omelet
Per serving: calories 277; fat 16.5 g; fiber 5 g; protein 20 g; carbohydrates 13 g

My old standby favorite got a delicious make-over for this book. I added avocado to leave you glowing and beautiful all day long. This is a great way to add vegetables to your breakfast; the Manly Beer Chili is packed full of metabolism-boosting veggies and makes this skinny, healthy breakfast taste too good to be true.

If you don't have any homemade chili on hand, canned organic low-sodium vegetarian chili will do in a pinch, but make sure to read the label and especially the ingredients list to ensure that the chili is low sodium and all natural. Many inexpensive canned chilis are packed full of sodium and chemical-derived thickening agents, which will leave you bloated while hindering your weight-loss efforts.

½ cup Manly Beer Chili (page 196)
Olive oil spray
2 large eggs
2 egg whites
4 tablespoons shredded sharp cheddar
  cheese
½ avocado, pitted, peeled, and sliced

1. In a medium saucepan, reheat the chili over medium-low heat.

2. Heat a small skillet over medium heat and spray it lightly with olive oil.

3. In a medium bowl, whisk together 1 egg, 1 egg white, and ½ teaspoon water. Add the egg mixture to the hot skillet and cook, undisturbed, until the eggs start to bubble on top. Add 2 tablespoons of the cheese, sprinkling it over one side of the omelet, then flip the other side over the cheese to make a half-moon. Cook for 2 minutes, then flip and cook for 2 minutes more, or until the cheese has melted and the eggs are firm. Transfer the omelet to a plate. Repeat to make the second omelet.

4. Top the omelets with hot chili and sliced avocado and serve.

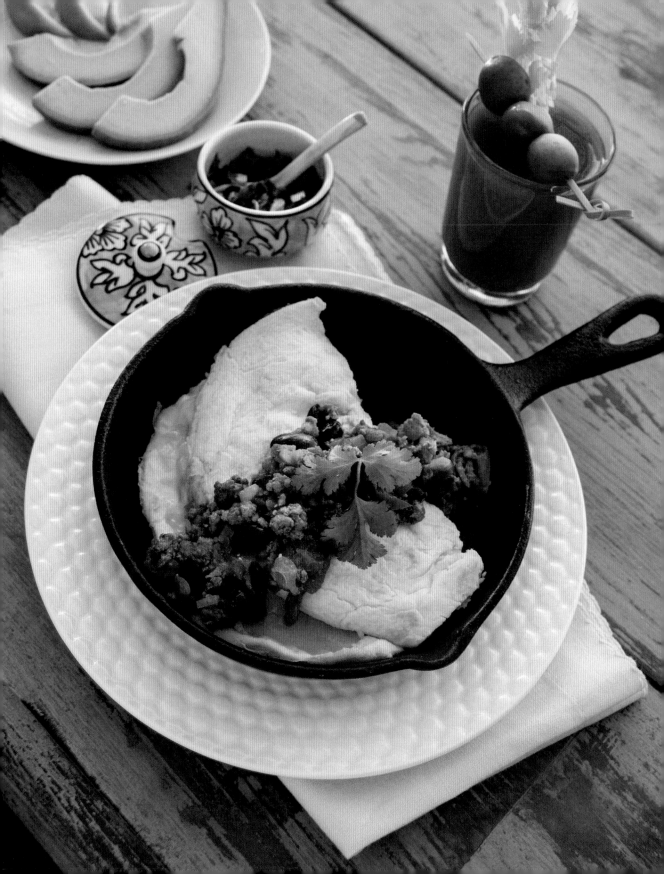

Breakfast Scramble

Makes 6 servings
Serving size: ⅓ cup veggie mixture, 1 egg, and 2 tablespoons cheese
Per serving: calories 194; fat 8 g; fiber 2 g; protein 14 g; carbohydrates 15 g

I used to buy frozen bags of breakfast scramble for camping trips and overnight houseguests, and I never realized how overpriced they were until I made my own. I chop up the veggies, add them to a gallon freezer bag, and pop it in the freezer. For fast weekday meals I grab a cup of the mixture and toss it in a pan and sauté it up while I make sack lunches. I add three eggs and a sprinkling of cheese and I've got a healthy, stick-to-your-ribs breakfast for three people in just fifteen minutes.

Make it easy on yourself: add a ⅓-cup measuring cup to your frozen bag of breakfast scramble and leave it in there!

1 large russet potato, peeled
1 jalapeño
1 yellow onion
1 red bell pepper
6 turkey or chicken breakfast sausage links
Olive oil spray
Kosher salt and freshly ground
    black pepper
6 large eggs
Hot sauce (optional)
¼ cup grated sharp cheddar or
    Gruyère cheese, or a combo of both
Handful of fresh cilantro, chopped
    (optional)

1. Chop the potato into very small cubes, the size of the tip of your pinkie finger. Place in a microwave-safe plate or bowl and microwave for 2½ minutes. Set aside to cool.

2. Slice the jalapeño in half lengthwise and remove the seeds and ribs (this will make it less spicy).

3. Chop the jalapeño, onion, bell pepper, and sausages into cubes the same size as the potato. (You can freeze everything in a gallon freezer bag at this stage if you like.)

4. Heat a large skillet over medium-high heat and lightly spray it with olive oil.

5. Add the veggies, potato, and sausage to the hot skillet, and add a dash of salt and pepper. Cook, stirring often to prevent burning, for about 10 minutes. When the potato is browned, the onion is soft, and the sausage is cooked through, reduce the heat to medium-low and push the cooked veggies and sausage to the outer rim of the pan.

6. In a medium bowl, whisk the eggs (if you like a spicy scramble, add a couple dashes of hot sauce). Pour the eggs into the center of the pan and use a wooden spoon to scramble the eggs, gently scraping the bottom of the pan as you go. Once the eggs start to set, mix in the veggies and sausage, turn off the heat, sprinkle with cheese, and cover. Let sit, covered, with the heat off for 3 minutes as the eggs finish cooking and the cheese melts. Serve topped with the cilantro, if using, and enjoy.

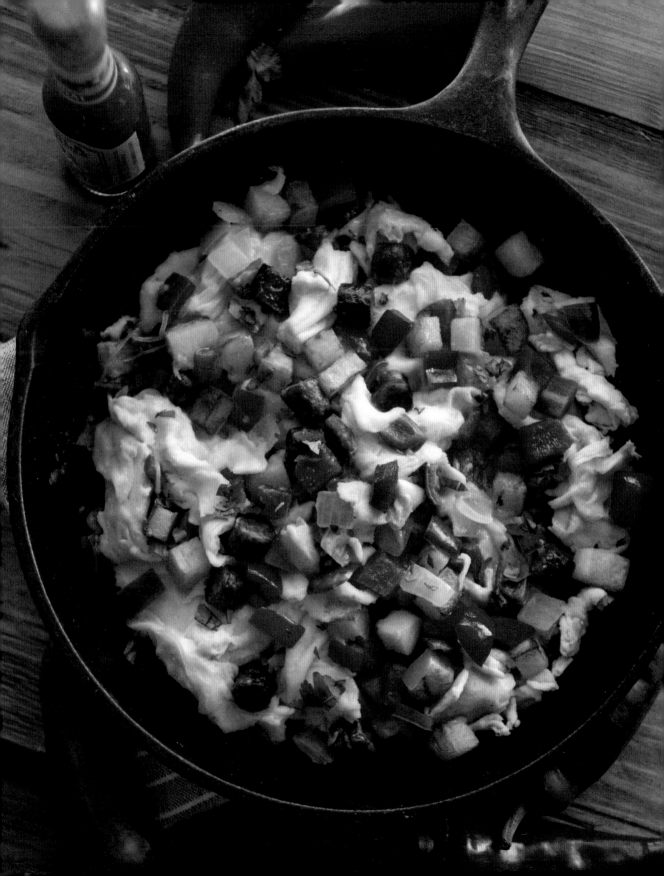

Chapter 3

The Best of Baked Goods

There's so much demonization of carbohydrates and sweets these days. Of course there are good and bad carbohydrates and sweets, but it's the bad carbs that are giving the good carbs a bad name. I want to help lift the veil on this myth. You *can* lose weight while eating bread and sweets. It's all in the ingredients you use. You hear on the news that sugar is causing most of the world's health issues, but have you taken into account what they are talking about? Kids don't drink milk nowadays, they drink chocolate milk; people don't eat veggies and fruits as snacks, they eat cookies and ice cream. The sugar epidemic is real, but it's no reason to throw the baby out with the bathwater.

First off, you want to opt for organic whenever possible. Most organic flours and sugars are less processed, full of nutrition, and contain fewer pesticides. Second, pay attention to the serving sizes. Remember, all things in moderation. Finally, use Smart Swaps whenever possible. Instead of substituting chemicals (fake sugars) for sugar, swap in all-natural honey or maple syrup or, better yet, mashed fruits. Remember how silly we all felt when we found out the fat-free diet of the 1990s was BS? Keep that in mind when it comes to weight-loss fads.

My favorite Smart Swaps for this chapter:

Applesauce works well in place of butter and sugar.

Greek yogurt is a good substitute for butter and oil, plus it adds creaminess and protein.

Almond milk adds sweetness, and at only 60 calories per cup it cuts a lot of calories from recipes.

Chocolate Chip Muffins

Makes 24 muffins
Serving size: 1 muffin
Per serving: calories 93; fat 3 g; fiber 1 g; protein 2.5 g; carbohydrates 16 g

When I look up healthy muffin recipes in cookbooks, the first thing I look for is the size of the muffin, so I want to tell you up front that these are indeed full-size muffins, not mini muffins. For those of you who prefer mini muffins, drop the baking time to 8 to 10 minutes and use mini chocolate chips or chop up standard chips.

I swapped in Greek yogurt and applesauce for the butter and half the sugar, cutting hundreds of calories and adding loads of moisture for super-fluffy muffins.

Olive oil spray
1½ cups self-rising flour
1 teaspoon baking soda
¼ teaspoon kosher salt
½ cup packed brown sugar
3 large eggs
1 teaspoon pure vanilla extract
¾ cup 0% Greek yogurt
½ cup unsweetened almond milk
½ cup Homemade Applesauce (page 112)
¾ cup semisweet chocolate chips

1. Preheat the oven to 350°F. Spray a muffin pan with olive oil (if you plan to use paper liners, spray the insides with olive oil as well).

2. In a large bowl, combine the flour, baking soda, salt, and sugar. Set aside.

3. In a medium bowl, whisk together the eggs, vanilla, Greek yogurt, almond milk, and applesauce.

4. Pour the wet ingredients into the dry ingredients and add the chocolate chips, reserving a handful to top the muffins. Fold the wet and dry ingredients together until just combined. Don't overmix, or you'll have tough muffins.

5. Fill the prepared muffin cups three-quarters full of batter and dot the tops with the remaining chocolate chips. Bake for 15 minutes, or until a toothpick inserted into the center of a muffin comes out clean.

Blueberry Muffins: Swap in dried blueberries for the chocolate chips.

Chocolate Coconut Muffins: Top the muffins with unsweetened flaked coconut before baking.

Cranberry Orange Muffins: Substitute dried cranberries and the zest of 1 orange for the chocolate chips.

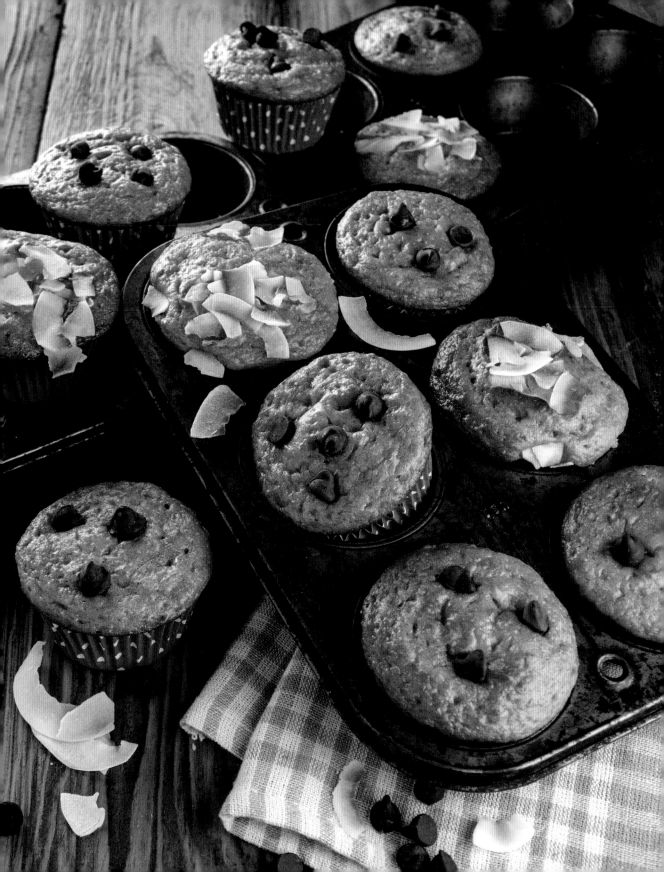

Strawberries and Cream Cookies

Makes 30 cookies
Serving size: 1 cookie
Per serving: calories 87; fat 2 g; fiber 1 g; protein 1 g; carbohydrates 16 g

I always loved those fruit-and-cream-flavored oatmeal packets when I was a kid, but now that I know they're full of preservatives and other chemicals that can cause weight gain, I have to get my fix elsewhere. So imagine my excitement when I found freeze-dried strawberries at my local health store. I finally had that one ingredient I needed to mimic my old favorite oatmeal packet: strawberries and cream. I have a popular Healthy Peaches and Cream Oatmeal Cookie recipe on my blog; this new take on that fan favorite is even easier, as you don't have to chop the dried fruit like you do in the original.

This is what I like to call a base recipe, because you can substitute other things for the strawberries and white chocolate—check out the variations opposite. You can even divide the batter into a few bowls and add different flavors to each.

¾ cup all-purpose flour
½ teaspoon baking soda
¼ teaspoon sea salt
2 tablespoons unsalted butter,
    at room temperature
1 cup packed light brown sugar
1 large egg
1 teaspoon pure vanilla extract
½ cup Homemade Applesauce (page 112)
2 cups old-fashioned rolled oats
½ cup white chocolate chips
½ cup chopped dried strawberries

1. In a medium bowl, combine the flour, baking soda, and salt.

2. In a large bowl or the bowl of a stand mixer fitted with the paddle attachment, whip the butter and sugar until pale and fluffy. Whisk in the egg and vanilla, then whisk in the applesauce and ⅓ cup water.

3. Slowly stir the flour mixture into the wet mixture until just combined. Fold in the oats, white chocolate chips, and strawberries. Cover the bowl and refrigerate the dough for 15 minutes to firm it up.

4. Meanwhile, preheat the oven to 350°F. Line two rimmed baking sheets with parchment paper.

5. Scoop Ping-Pong-ball-size dollops of cookie dough onto the prepared baking sheets, leaving 1½ inches between them to allow for a little spreading. Bake for 10 to 15 minutes, or until the cookies are golden brown. Transfer to a wire rack to cool for softer cookies, or leave on the baking sheet to cool for crispier cookies.

NOTE: For homemade Strawberries and Cream Oatmeal, see page 25.

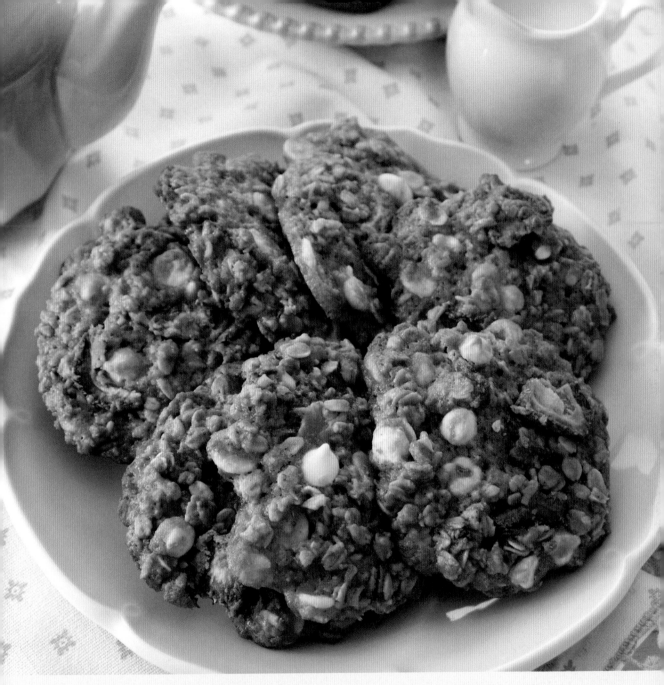

Dark Chocolate Cherry: Substitute ½ cup dark chocolate chips and ½ cup dried cherries for the strawberries and white chocolate.

Peaches and Cream: Swap in ½ cup chopped dried peaches for the strawberries.

Chocolate Chip: Use ½ cup dark chocolate chips in place of the strawberries and white chocolate.

Blueberries and Cream: Substitute ½ cup dried blueberries for the strawberries.

Lemon Almond Biscotti

Makes 16 cookies
Serving size: 1 cookie
Per serving: calories 66; fat 1 g; fiber .5 g; protein 1.5 g; carbohydrates 12.5 g

These bright lemon cookies are packed with flavor. Try them dipped in a Vanilla Latte (page 268). They're great little gifts for new neighbors and teachers, and they're perfect for selling at bake sales. If you want to jazz them up a bit, dip half of each cookie in melted white chocolate and sprinkle with crushed almonds. Gifts are all about presentation—place the biscotti in clear gift bags wrapped in pretty ribbon or 3-cup mason jars with colorful fabric swatches.

P.S. Santa also loves these, and kids love to help bake them.

1 cup all-purpose flour
¼ cup chopped almonds
¾ teaspoon baking powder
¼ teaspoon kosher salt
Zest of 2 lemons
1 large egg
½ cup sugar
1 teaspoon pure vanilla extract
2 tablespoons fresh lemon juice

1. Preheat the oven to 350°F. Line a baking sheet with parchment paper.

2. In a medium bowl, combine the flour, almonds, baking powder, salt, and lemon zest.

3. In the bowl of a stand mixer fitted with the paddle attachment or in a large bowl, beat the egg and sugar on medium speed until thick and pale, about 5 minutes. Reduce the speed to low and add the vanilla and lemon juice. Slowly add the flour mixture and mix until just combined; do not overmix, or you'll end up with tough cookies.

4. Transfer the dough to the prepared baking sheet. With wet hands, mold the dough into one large rectangular block about a foot long. Bake for about 20 minutes, until slightly browned around the edges.

5. Remove the baking sheet from the oven (but leave the oven on) and let the block cool for 10 minutes.

6. Move the block to a cutting board and carefully remove the parchment paper from the bottom. Cut the block crosswise into ½-inch cookies and set them back on the parchment paper–lined baking sheet, cut side up. Bake for 10 minutes, turning the cookies over halfway through, until golden brown.

7. Let the cookies cool completely on a wire rack. They will crisp up more as they cool!

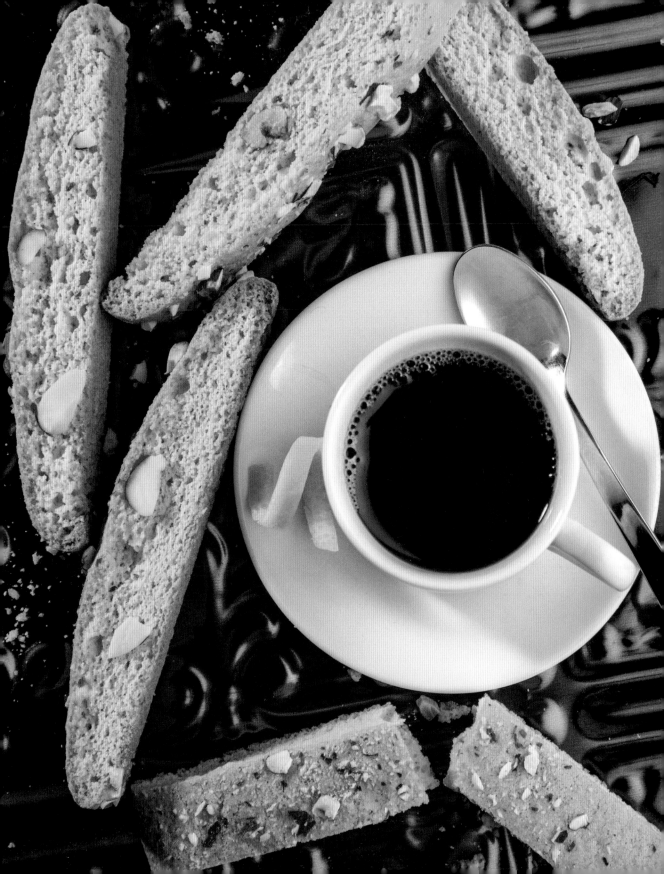

Dark Chocolate Fudge Brownies

Makes 21 brownies
Serving size: 1 brownie
Per serving: calories 108; fat 4.5 g; fiber 1 g; protein 3 g; carbohydrates 16 g

I absolutely love chocolate, but, being a purist to the core, I just can't bring myself to use ingredients like black beans in my brownies. I make these fudgy brownies when the craving comes, and to be honest, the craving comes often. They're rich and decadent without being tooth-achingly sweet, and best of all, the cleanup is easy. You just make the batter in a saucepan, dump it into a casserole dish, and bake!

4 tablespoons (½ stick) unsalted butter
1 cup semisweet chocolate chips
½ cup packed dark brown sugar
1 cup 0% Greek yogurt
1 teaspoon pure vanilla extract
2 large eggs
1 teaspoon baking soda
½ cup unsweetened cocoa powder
1¼ cups all-purpose flour

1. Preheat the oven to 350°F. Line a 9 x 13-inch baking dish with parchment paper.

2. In a large saucepan, melt the butter, chocolate chips, and sugar over medium heat until smooth. Set aside to cool slightly, about 5 minutes, or until warm.

3. Whisk in the Greek yogurt and vanilla and let the mixture cool to room temperature. Add the eggs and whisk to combine.

4. Whisk in the baking soda, cocoa powder, and flour until you have a smooth, mousse-like batter.

5. Scrape the batter into the prepared baking dish and smooth it to the edges so that the top is level. Bake for 25 to 30 minutes, or until the top is firm to the touch.

6. Let the brownies cool completely in the pan, about 30 minutes, then pull up on the parchment paper and transfer them to a cutting board. Peel the paper away and use a sharp knife to cut them into twenty-one squares (two long cuts and six short cuts).

Make these into brownie bites: Spray mini-muffin pans with olive oil spray. Spoon the batter into the pans. Bake for 10 to 15 minutes and cool for 10 minutes before serving.

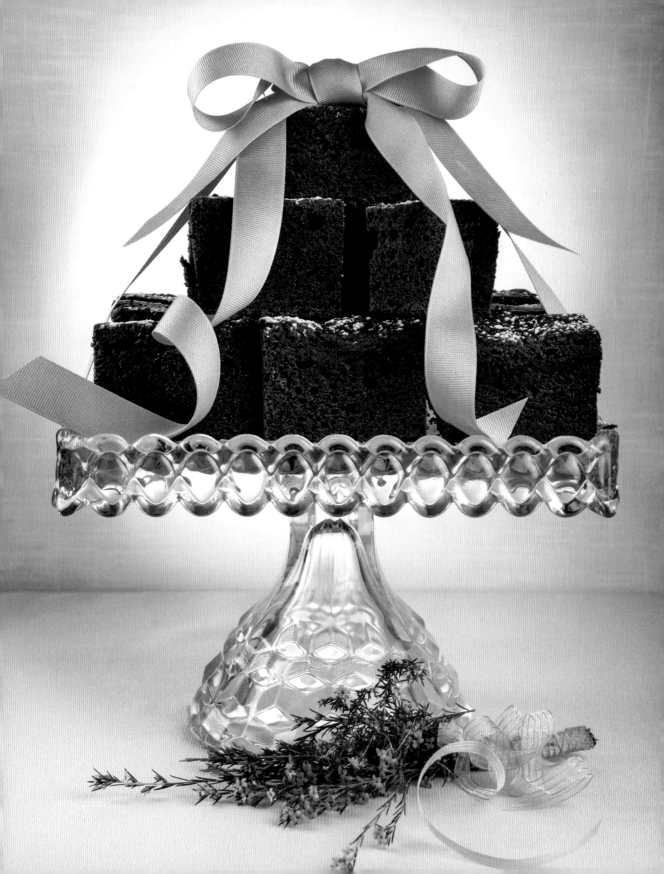

The White and Wheat Combo Loaf

Makes 1 large loaf (about 20 slices)
Serving size: 1 slice
Per serving: calories 78; fat 1 g; fiber 2 g; protein 2.5 g; carbohydrates 15 g

I typically make an all-wheat loaf, and you can easily swap in more wheat here, but this recipe is for everyone who's trying to get his or her family on board with a healthier lifestyle. This combo loaf gets kids used to a heartier bread. As time progresses, add more wheat flour and omit more white flour until you have a wheat to white ratio you're happy with.

I love making my own bread because I know what's in it and can be sure that all the nasty preservatives and other chemicals never make it to my family's plates. If you've never made bread before, don't fret—it's easy and very gratifying making your first loaf, so be brave and dive in!

2 cups wheat flour
1½ cups all-purpose flour
1 tablespoon kosher salt
1 packet Fleischmann's RapidRise Yeast
2 cups warm water
1 tablespoon olive oil

1. In the bowl of a stand mixer or a large bowl, combine the flours, salt, and yeast. Add 1 cup of the warm water and mix with a spatula. Gradually add the remaining 1 cup water and the olive oil and mix until the ingredients come together and start to resemble a ball of dough.

2. If you're using a stand mixer, put on the dough hook attachment and mix on medium speed for 5 minutes. If not, turn the dough out onto a clean, floured surface and knead by hand for 5 minutes. Your dough should be slightly warm and smooth to the touch.

3. Flour the inside of the mixing bowl and drop in the kneaded dough. Cover with plastic wrap and a kitchen towel and place in a warm spot to rise for 1 to 3 hours. You know it is ready when it's doubled in size.

4. Punch down the dough to deflate it. Give it a quick 1-minute knead, then shape it on a baking sheet or in a standard-size loaf pan. Re-cover the shaped dough with the plastic wrap and the kitchen towel and let it rise for another 30 minutes, or until doubled in size again.

5. When the dough is almost risen, preheat the oven to 425°F.

6. Remove the towel and plastic wrap and bake the bread for 30 to 35 minutes, until golden brown on the top and around the edges. To test that the bread is fully baked, gently flip the bread or remove it from the loaf pan to expose the bottom (protect your hands—keep your oven mitts on). Knock on the bottom of the loaf with a wooden spoon—if it sounds hollow, the bread is done. Let cool completely, then slice with a serrated knife.

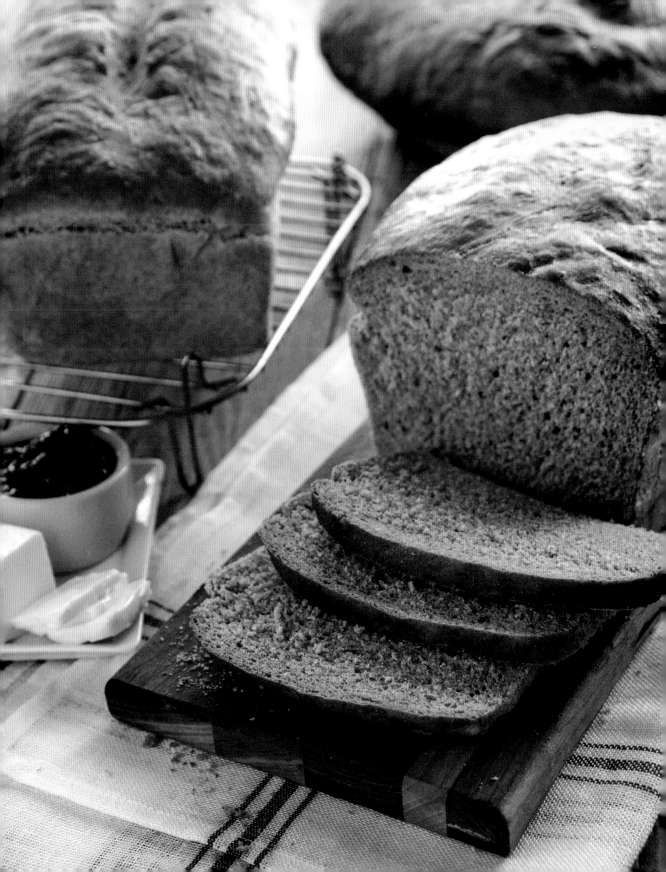

Garlic Bread

Makes 1 loaf (about 16 slices)
Serving size: 1 slice
Per serving: calories 57; fat 2.5 g; fiber 0 g; protein 1.5 g; carbohydrates 6 g

I love this garlic bread recipe because you can make it many different ways—with sliced bread, on a large French roll, on mini baguettes, on almost any bread you have in the house. I've tried it all! I recommend using a long, wide loaf of French bread from the bakery section of your grocery store.

If sixteen servings is too many, you can prep the whole loaf and bake just half. Wrap the other half in waxed paper, place in a freezer bag, and freeze. You'll have garlic bread ready to bake just waiting in your freezer. You can defrost it in the fridge before baking, or toss it in the oven straight from the freezer (just add 10 minutes to your bake time).

2 heads garlic, unpeeled
1 tablespoon olive oil
Kosher salt and freshly ground
    black pepper
2 tablespoons unsalted butter, cold
3 tablespoons freshly grated
    Parmesan cheese
1 loaf French bread

1. Preheat the oven to 350°F. Tear off a 2-foot piece of aluminum foil.

2. Cut the top third from each garlic head, revealing the tops of the garlic cloves. Place the garlic heads on the foil, drizzle with the olive oil, and sprinkle lightly with salt and pepper. Wrap the foil around the heads to make a loose but well-sealed packet. Place the foil packet in an oven-safe dish to catch any spillage and roast the garlic for 1 hour, or until the garlic cloves pop out easily and are extremely soft. Leave the oven on.

3. Let the garlic cool before removing it from the foil packet. When the garlic is cool enough to handle, pour all the hot oil in a shallow bowl and use a fork to help slide the garlic cloves into the bowl with the oil.

4. Use the back of a fork to smash the garlic cloves until they're mush. Add the butter and smash until combined. Mix in the grated cheese.

5. Slice the bread in half lengthwise and place it on a baking sheet, cut side up.

6. Spoon half the garlic mixture onto each bread half and smooth it out evenly. Bake for 8 to 15 minutes, until the cheese starts to brown.

7. Remove from the oven and let cool slightly, 3 to 5 minutes, before cutting with a serrated knife or sharp kitchen scissors. Cut each loaf half into eight slices. Start by cutting the loaf in half, then cut each of those halves in half and then again, like you're cutting a sushi roll. This will help keep all the portions even.

NOTE: You can add this bread in with whatever else you've got cooking in the oven if it's set anywhere between 325°F and 450°F—just watch carefully so it doesn't burn. At lower temperatures, the bread will need longer in the oven; in hotter ovens it will need less time.

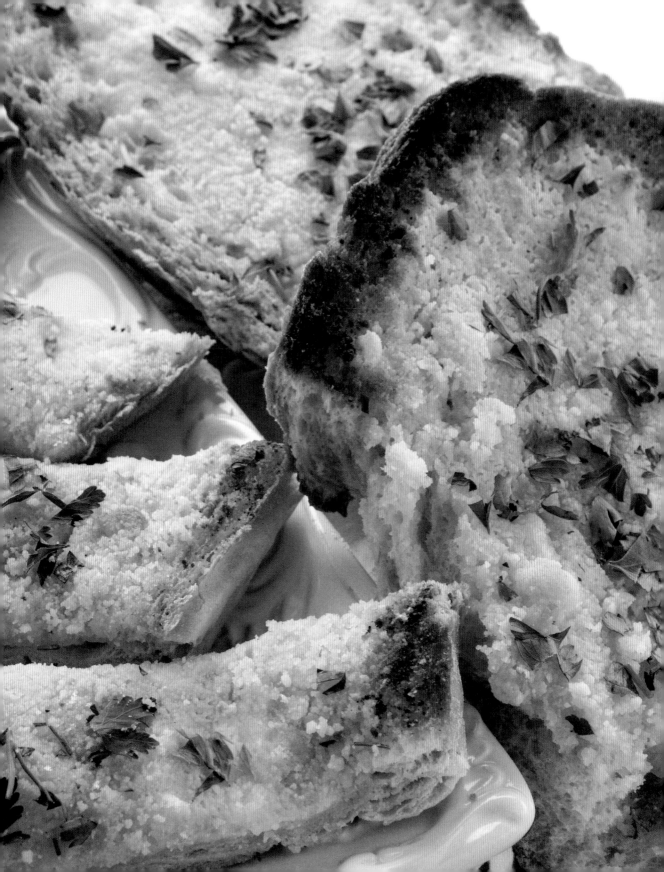

Jalapeño Cheddar Scones

Makes 16 scones
Serving size: 1 scone
Per serving: calories 126; fat 3.5 g; fiber 1 g; protein 4 g; carbohydrates 19 g

These scones are great for dinner parties—skip rolls and serve these instead. They're a hit for any occasion, from a barbecue to an elegant dinner party.

I often make these along with the Strawberry Scones with Lime Glaze (page 60) for brunch or tea, giving my guests more to choose from and impressing them with my baking skills.

3 jalapeños
3 cups all-purpose flour
1 teaspoon baking powder
1 teaspoon baking soda
2 teaspoons kosher salt
3 tablespoons unsalted butter, cold
¾ cup unsweetened almond milk
½ cup 0% Greek yogurt
½ cup shredded sharp cheddar cheese

1. Preheat the oven to 375°F. Line a rimmed baking sheet with parchment paper.

2. Slice 2 of the jalapeños lengthwise into four pieces each. Using a small knife, scrape out and discard the seeds and ribs. Dice the jalapeños and set aside. Slice the remaining jalapeño into thin rings and remove the seeds and ribs. Set aside.

3. In a large bowl or the bowl of a stand mixer fitted with the paddle attachment, beat together the flour, baking powder, baking soda, and salt. Cut the butter into small pieces and add it to the flour mixture. Work the flour and butter together with your fingers until the butter is in chunks the size of peas (if you're using a stand mixer, you should still do this part by hand).

4. In a medium bowl, whisk together the almond milk and Greek yogurt. Pour half the yogurt mixture into the flour mixture and fold it in. Add the rest of the yogurt mixture, the diced jalapeños, and the cheese, reserving some cheese to top the scones. Mix gently until incorporated, but do not overmix or the scones will be tough.

5. Divide the dough in half and place the dough balls on a floured surface. Squish and mold them into two foot-long rectangles. Use a pizza wheel to slice each rectangle once lengthwise and four times across into eight equal squares.

6. Arrange the scones on the prepared baking sheet; they can be close together, but don't let them touch. Top each scone with a little cheese and a jalapeño ring. Bake for 13 to 16 minutes, or until slightly golden.

For an hors d'oeuvre–size scone, make three dough balls and cut eight scones from each for twenty-four scones total. Bake for 10 to 13 minutes.

For mild, kid-friendly heat, make some scones without jalapeño rings on top.

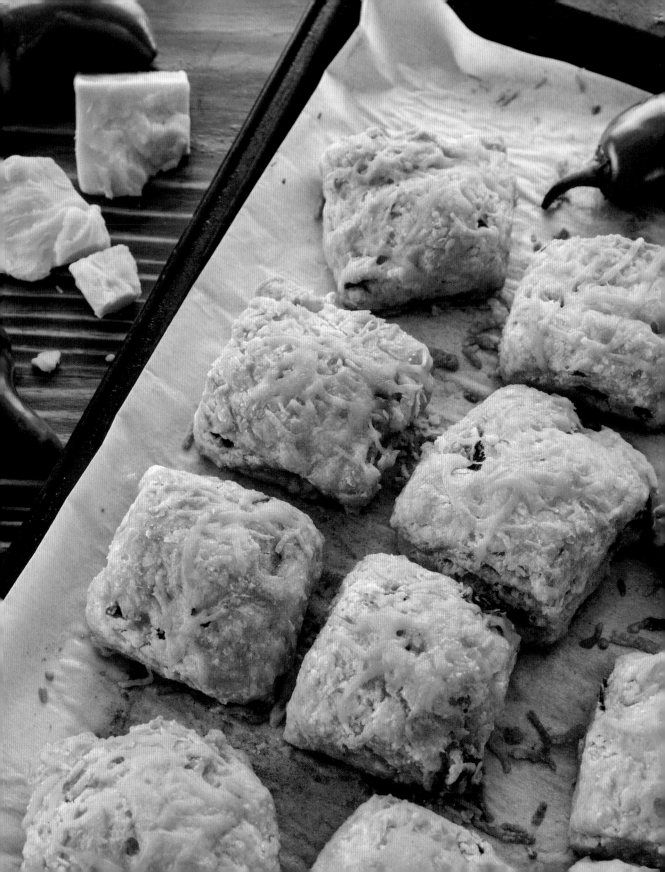

Strawberry Scones with Lime Glaze

Makes 16 scones
Serving size: 1 scone
Per serving: calories 149; fat 2.5 g; fiber 1 g; protein 2.5 g; carbohydrates 28 g

My favorite local coffee shop gets the most amazing bakery goods fresh each morning. One day, the barista convinced me to try the newest goodie: strawberry, lime, and basil scones. They were delicious, and I was inspired to make a healthy, low-calorie version at home. As I worked on the recipe, the basil was omitted. You can try it yourself, but I find the lime zest gives a brighter flavor. I cut calories by swapping in almond milk for buttermilk and using applesauce in place of half the sugar and butter.

You can find dried strawberries on online grocery websites like Amazon and Thrive Market, or try dried cranberries or pineapple or your favorite unsweetened dried fruit.

Scones

3 cups all-purpose flour
¼ cup granulated sugar
1 teaspoon baking powder
1 teaspoon baking soda
Zest of 3 limes
4 tablespoons (½ stick) unsalted butter, cold
¾ cup unsweetened almond milk
½ cup Homemade Applesauce (page 112)
½ cup chopped dried strawberries

Glaze

½ cup powdered sugar
3 teaspoons lime juice, plus more
    as needed

1. Make the scones: Preheat the oven to 375°F. Line a rimmed baking sheet with parchment paper.

2. In a large bowl or the bowl of a stand mixer fitted with the paddle attachment, beat the flour, sugar, baking powder, baking soda, and lime zest. Cut the butter into small pieces and add it to the flour. Work the flour and butter together with your fingers until the butter is in chunks the size of peas (if you're using a stand mixer, you should still do this part by hand).

3. In a medium bowl, whisk together the almond milk and applesauce. Pour half the applesauce mixture into the flour mixture and stir to combine. Add the rest of the applesauce mixture and the strawberries and mix gently until incorporated, but do not overmix or the scones will be tough.

4. Divide the dough in half and place the dough balls on a floured surface. Squish and mold them into two discs about 6 inches across. Use a pizza wheel to slice each disc into eight equal triangles, as if you're cutting a pizza or a pie.

5. Arrange the scones on the prepared baking sheet; they can be close together, but don't let them touch. Bake for 13 to 16 minutes, until golden on top. Transfer the scones to a wire rack to cool completely before adding the glaze.

6. Make the glaze: Sift the powdered sugar into a small bowl. Slowly add ½ teaspoon of the lime juice at a time until the glaze is just runny enough to drizzle off your spoon. Drizzle the glaze over the cooled scones and let it set for 30 minutes before serving.

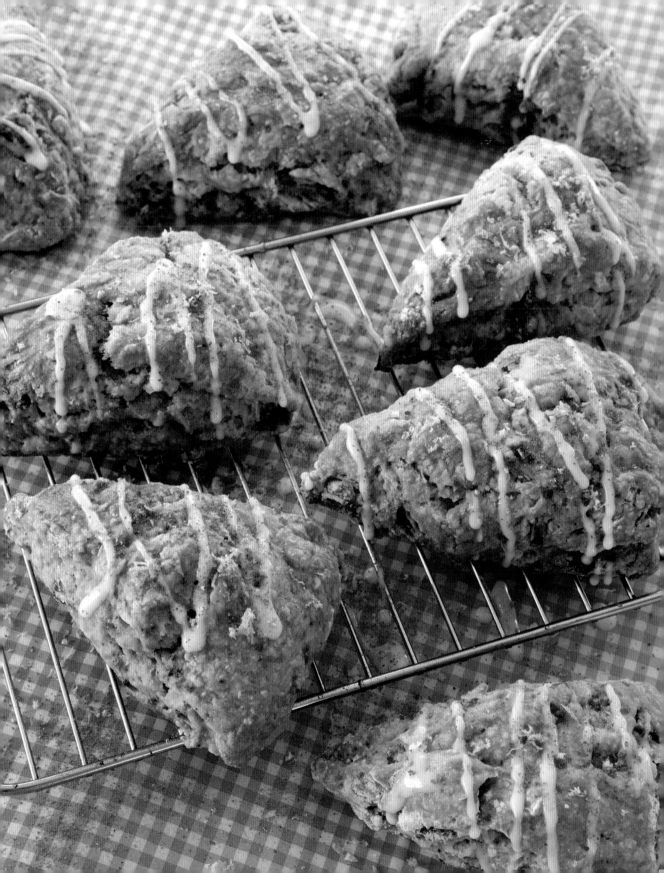

Chapter 4

Between Two Pieces of Bread

There are few meals easier and more satisfying than a good sandwich. Fancy food trucks are popping up with decadent meals squished between two slices of bread. They're simple, inexpensive, and travel well—no wonder they're so popular!

In this chapter I wanted to give you lots of sandwich options, from five easy-to-make panini (without a panini maker!) to sliders, hoagies, and even a wrap. Your lunch box will never be boring again, and you may even find yourself making these for a fast, no-fuss dinner.

My favorite Smart Swaps for this chapter:

Sharp cheese has more flavor than mild, so you can use less and get the same flavor punch.

Whole wheat bread has more nutrients than bleached white, and it gives you loads of healthy fiber to keep you full for hours.

Greek yogurt adds moisture and creaminess without all the fat of mayonnaise.

Panini a Day: Five Panini Recipes

Grown-up grilled cheese has become a phenomenon. Fancy food trucks and storefronts specialize in them, and upscale restaurants are adding chic ingredients, calling them panini, and charging a fortune. These panini are inspired by food (sandwiches and other things!) at the amazing food trucks and tiny restaurants I've had the pleasure to dine at.

Here's a secret: you can make these upscale grilled cheese sandwiches for a fraction of the price, half the calories, and triple the nutrition—and you don't even need a panini maker. All you need is a grated griddle or pan and another heavy, slightly smaller pan. Use the smaller pan to squish down the sandwich and voilà—you've got a homemade panini maker. If you do have a panini maker (lucky!), just follow the manufacturer's instructions when it comes to cooking the sandwiches.

These impressive sandwiches are great for easy yet impressive weekend lunches and wonderful for dinner with a cup of soup (try the Chicken Tortilla Soup on page 182) or a crisp salad (see page 18 for ideas).

NOTE: If you're more of a grilled cheese fan, you can make all these recipes as grilled cheeses. Use a smooth pan instead of a grated one, and cover with a lid to help melt the cheese.

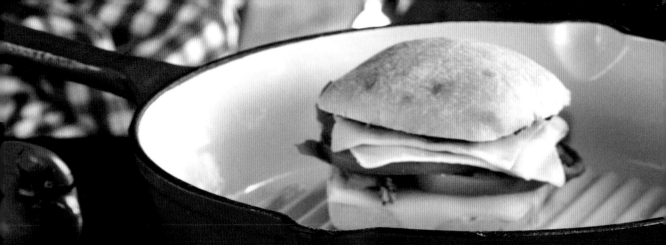

Avocado Chicken Panini, page 69

Pesto Chicken Panini, page 71

Tomato Basil Mozzarella Panini, page 66

Tomato Basil Mozzarella Panini

Makes 2 panini
Serving size: 1 sandwich
Per serving: calories 284; fat 4.5 g; fiber 4.5 g; protein 13 g; carbohydrates 47 g

I often eat vegetarian meals for breakfast and lunch, and later I'll make a family-friendly chicken or steak dinner. I feel better when I eat this way, and I save money as well—bonus! This is one of those go-to meals for my vegetarian lunches. If you feel you need a protein boost, add some shredded or sliced cooked chicken breast.

For this sandwich I buy a ball of fresh mozzarella and slice it myself. I love the ooze you get from a thick slice of the stark white cheese, but you can use shredded mozzarella as well. If your mozzarella ball is too soft to slice easily, freeze it for an hour. You can slice the entire ball or slice what you need now and shred the rest for pizza (see chapter 7).

2 teaspoons Skinny Pesto (page 71)
4 slices whole wheat sourdough bread
1 tomato, sliced
8 to 10 fresh basil leaves
2 (¼-inch-thick) slices fresh mozzarella, or ¼ cup shredded mozzarella
Olive oil spray

1. Smear 1 teaspoon of the pesto on each of 2 slices of bread and top with the tomato, basil, mozzarella, and the remaining slices of bread.

2. Lightly spray both sides of the sandwiches with olive oil spray.

3. Heat a grill pan or griddle over medium heat or preheat a panini maker. Place the sandwiches in the hot pan and push down on them with the bottom of a small, heavy pan (or cook the sandwiches in the panini maker according to the manufacturer's instructions). Cook for 5 minutes. When one side is browned, flip the sandwiches, press down again with the top pan, and cook for 3 to 5 minutes, or until the bread is browned and the cheese is oozing.

4. Slice the sandwiches in half and serve.

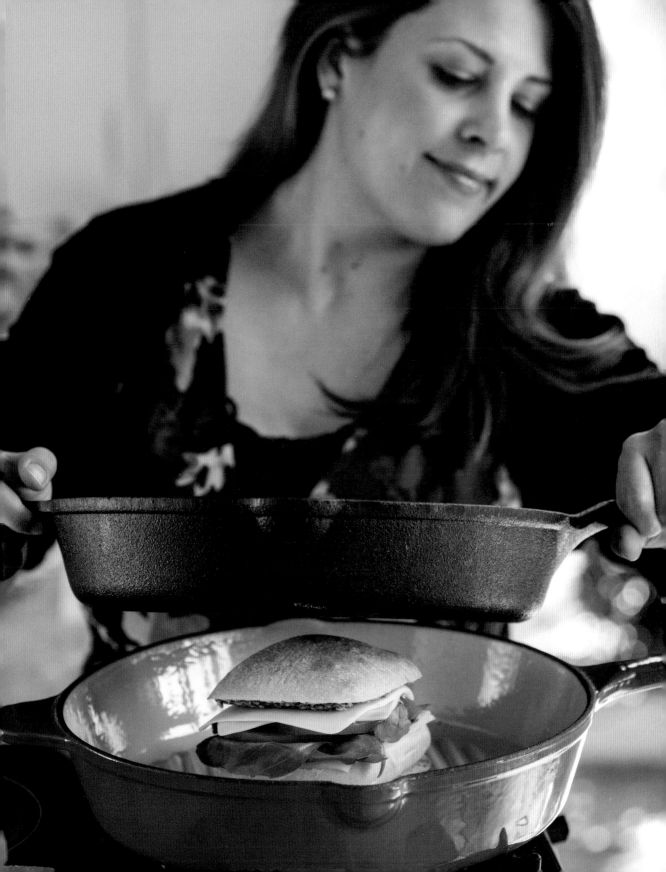

Elvis-Inspired Grilled Peanut Butter Banana Panini

Makes 2 panini
Serving size: 1 sandwich
Per serving: calories 366; fat 10 g; fiber 6.5 g; protein 10 g; carbohydrates 61 g

---

The King inspired many artists with his music, but it was his love for food that inspired me! This sandwich is actually one of my favorite breakfasts, but I felt it fit better here in the panini section. Cut it into four triangles for fancy sleepover treats you can feel good about giving to your kiddos, or enjoy as a lunch that also helps curb your afternoon craving for sweets.

Go for all-natural, no-added-sugar peanut butter here—you want pure health, not over-processed, sugar-filled junk!

1 banana
4 slices whole wheat bread
2 tablespoons all-natural peanut butter
Olive oil spray

1. In a small bowl, smash the banana with the back of a fork. Smear it evenly on 2 slices of bread.

2. Smear 1 tablespoon of the peanut butter on each of the other 2 slices of bread. Lay the peanut butter sides on the banana sides and press together gently.

3. Lightly spray both sides of the sandwiches with olive oil.

4. Heat a grill pan or griddle over medium heat or preheat a panini maker. Place the sandwiches in the hot pan and push down on them with the bottom of a small, heavy pan (or cook the sandwiches in the panini maker according to the manufacturer's instructions). Cook for 5 minutes. When one side is browned, flip the sandwiches, press down again with the top pan and cook for 3 to 5 minutes, or until the bread is browned and the peanut butter is oozing.

5. Slice the sandwiches in half and serve.

There is a debate about which sandwich Elvis loved more, the peanut butter and banana sandwich or the peanut butter, banana, and *bacon* sandwich. If you want to try this panini with bacon, simply cook 1 slice bacon in the skillet, crumble the cooked bacon, and divide it between the panini. Also, skip the olive oil spray and instead use 2 teaspoons of the bacon drippings in the pan to cook the sandwiches. This will add about 100 calories per sandwich.

Avocado Chicken Panini

Makes 2 panini
Serving size: 1 sandwich
Per serving: calories 397; fat 12.5 g; fiber 6 g; protein 24 g; carbohydrates 47 g

---

I live in California, where avocados are in abundance all year round, but you can swap in tomato as needed or desired. This recipe is also great for using leftover chicken!

Don't be scared of the fat in this panini, as most of it comes from the avocado. Avocados contain good fats (unsaturated), and some studies have even shown that eating these good fats can help your body release fat faster, aiding in weight loss. Avocados are one of my favorite "beauty foods"; they make your skin glow, your nails stronger, and your hair shinier, and they also help lower cholesterol and inflammation and can aid your body in absorbing nutrients better, including fiber, which will keep you full longer.

Olive oil spray
1 boneless, skinless chicken breast
Kosher salt and freshly ground
    black pepper
½ ripe avocado, pitted, peeled, and diced
1 tablespoon Five-Minute Salsa (page 96)
    or your favorite salsa
⅓ cup shredded cheddar cheese
4 slices whole wheat sourdough bread

1. Heat a grated pan or griddle over medium heat. Lightly spray it with olive oil. Sprinkle the chicken breast with a pinch of salt and pepper, add it to the pan, and cook it for about 5 minutes on each side, until cooked through and browned. Reserve any juices in the pan for cooking the panini, and let the chicken cool for 10 minutes.

2. With a serrated knife, half the chicken breast horizontally to make two thin patties (or shred the chicken with two forks).

3. In a medium bowl, combine the avocado and salsa. Use a fork to smash the mixture together to the desired consistency (I like it chunky, but if you like it smooth, smash a little longer).

4. Time to put together the sandwiches! Sprinkle one-third of the cheese over 2 slices of bread, top with the chicken, sprinkle on half the remaining cheese, add the avocado mixture, and then sprinkle on the rest of the cheese. Top with the remaining slices of bread.

5. Heat the same pan in which you cooked the chicken over medium heat or preheat a panini maker. Place the sandwiches in the hot pan and push down on them with the bottom of a small, heavy pan (or cook the sandwiches in the panini maker according to the manufacturer's instructions). Cook for 5 minutes. When one side is browned, flip the sandwiches, press down again with the top pan, and cook for 3 to 5 minutes, or until the bread is browned and the cheese is oozing.

6. Slice the sandwiches in half and serve.

French Onion Grilled Panini

Makes 2 panini
Serving size: 1 sandwich
Per serving: calories 427; fat 11.5 g; fiber 4 g; protein 37 g; carbohydrates 46 g

Here's the thing about this sandwich—it's crazy delicious!

It's important that you get the nitrate-free, all-natural roast beef here. Most often that just means going to the deli counter, where you can find quality beef for the same price as the cheap, chemical-filled stuff that will only reverse your weight loss. If you have leftover steak, thinly slice it and use it in place of the roast beef; the "Everything" Rubbed Steaks (page 168) is especially yummy here.

This is a rich-tasting sandwich, so I usually serve it with a delicious crisp green salad with honey mustard vinaigrette. See my Guide to the Perfect Salad (page 18).

2 slices low-fat provolone, cut in half
4 slices sourdough or French bread
2 tablespoons Caramelized Onions
    (page 134)
4 slices fresh, nitrate-free deli roast beef
Olive oil spray

1. To assemble the sandwiches, layer 2 slices of bread with half a provolone slice each. Top each with 1 tablespoon of the caramelized onions, 2 slices of roast beef, the remaining cheese, and the remaining slices of bread. Press together and lightly spray both sides with olive oil spray.

2. Heat a grated pan or griddle over medium heat or preheat a panini maker. Place the sandwiches in the hot pan and push down on them with the bottom of a small, heavy pan (or cook the sandwiches in the panini maker according to the manufacturer's instructions). Cook for 5 minutes. When one side is browned, flip the sandwiches, press down again with the top pan, and cook for 3 to 5 minutes, or until the bread is browned and the cheese is oozing.

3. Slice the sandwiches in half and serve.

Pesto Chicken Panini

Makes 2 panini
Serving size: 1 sandwich
Per serving: calories 355; fat 8 g; fiber 4 g; protein 23 g; carbohydrates 44 g

I love this pesto sandwich, mainly because it packs tons of tastiness in just a few calories, which is the whole point of this book! Load up the flavor and nobody will notice that there's half the cheese and no butter. If you don't like pesto or want to change up this recipe, try some spicy brown or Dijon mustard in its place. Just like the pesto, it will boost the flavor without adding too many calories.

Swap avocado in for the chicken for a yummy vegetarian version!

Skinny Pesto

1 cup fresh basil leaves
1 tablespoon olive oil
2 tablespoons slivered almonds
1 clove garlic

Panini

Olive oil spray
1 boneless, skinless chicken breast
Kosher salt and freshly ground
    black pepper
2 tablespoons 0% Greek yogurt
4 slices whole wheat sourdough bread
⅓ cup shredded Gruyère or sharp cheddar
    cheese (or a combo of both)
8 to 10 fresh basil leaves
½ cup arugula

1. Make the Skinny Pesto: Combine all the ingredients in a food processor and process until smooth. Transfer the pesto to a small jar and store in the fridge for up to 1 week.

2. Make the panini: Heat a grill pan or griddle over medium heat. Spray it with olive oil. Sprinkle the chicken breast with salt and pepper, add it to the pan, and cook for about 5 minutes on each side, until browned and cooked through. Set the chicken aside to rest for 10 minutes and reserve the yummy drippings in the pan for cooking the panini.

3. Use a serrated knife to slice the chicken horizontally into two thin pieces.

4. In a small bowl, combine 2 teaspoons of the pesto and the Greek yogurt.

5. Smear each slice of bread with 2 teaspoons of the pesto-yogurt mixture. Sprinkle 2 slices with half the cheese and top with the chicken, basil leaves, and arugula (it will wilt, so don't be intimidated by the quantity). Add the rest of the cheese and top with the remaining bread.

6. Heat the pan you cooked the chicken in over medium heat or preheat a panini maker. Place the sandwiches in the hot pan and push down on them with the bottom of a small, heavy pan (or cook the sandwiches in the panini maker according to the manufacturer's instructions). Cook for 5 minutes. When one side is browned, flip the sandwiches, press down again with the top pan, and cook for 3 to 5 minutes, or until the bread is browned and the cheese is oozing.

7. Slice the sandwiches in half and serve.

Caesar Salad Wrap

Makes 4 wraps
Serving size: 1 wrap
Per serving: calories 292; fat 10.5 g; fiber 4.5 g; protein 15 g; carbohydrates 34 g

I had a favorite takeout place in my heavier days, and along with its amazing Caesar salad with chicken and rice (see loseweightbyeating .com for my skinny version), it made a divine Caesar salad wrap. I had to re-create it in a healthy way, and it was easy once I cracked the skinny dressing code. I used Smart Swaps like Greek yogurt and almond milk to cut the calories.

I know it may seem strange to put croutons in a wrap, but the crunch they offer in the soft wrap is too good to miss. Save your leftover bread and the heels of your loaves to make croutons. Just dedicate a large freezer bag for leftover bread and keep adding to it. You can also use these leftovers to make homemade bread crumbs (see Note, page 81), saving you money and trips to the store.

Dressing

½ cup 0% Greek yogurt
2 tablespoons unsweetened almond milk
2 tablespoons extra-virgin olive oil
¼ cup Dijon mustard
2 tablespoons balsamic vinegar
3 tablespoons fresh lemon juice
1 clove garlic, finely chopped
Kosher salt and freshly ground black pepper

Croutons

1 slice whole wheat sourdough or whole wheat bread
1 teaspoon olive oil
½ teaspoon garlic salt
Freshly ground black pepper (optional)

Wraps

2 romaine hearts, chopped
1 cup baby spinach, chopped
1 chicken breast, cooked and shredded
4 (8-inch) spinach or whole wheat wraps
1 avocado, sliced

1. Make the dressing: At least 1 hour ahead of time and up to 24 hours beforehand, in a medium jar or bowl, combine all the dressing ingredients. If using a jar, close the lid and shake well; if using a bowl, whisk together well and cover with plastic wrap. Refrigerate until it's time to assemble the wraps.

2. Make the croutons: Preheat the oven to 400°F. Cut the bread into small squares. In a large bowl, toss the bread cubes with the olive oil, garlic salt, and pepper, if using. Spread the cubes on a rimmed baking sheet and bake for 8 minutes, or until crispy and golden.

3. Make the salad: In the bowl you used for the croutons, combine the romaine, spinach, chicken, croutons, and two-thirds of the dressing. Toss until the salad is well coated with the dressing; add more dressing to taste.

4. To assemble the wraps, divide the salad evenly among the wraps and top with avocado slices. Wrap like a burrito, slice in half, and serve.

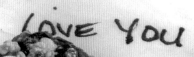

... BABY.
YOU ROCK MY
WORLD!

LOVE YOU

Nutty Chicken Salad Sliders

Makes 5 sliders
Serving size: 1 slider
Per serving: calories 151; fat 4.5 g; fiber 1.5 g; protein 10 g; carbohydrates 17 g

Just as with the French Bread Pizza (page 142), I cut these slider rolls in thirds and remove the middle third of the bread, thus removing a third of the carbs. What you want to do is cut off the top of the roll, then cut off the bottom, and save the inside for croutons (see page 72) or bread crumbs (see page 81). This will instantly save you tons of calories that you'll never miss.

1 chicken breast, cooked and chopped
   (see Note)
1 teaspoon dried cranberries, chopped
1½ teaspoons chopped pecans
½ red bell pepper, chopped
½ shallot, chopped
1½ teaspoons spicy brown or Dijon mustard
¼ cup 0% Greek yogurt
Kosher salt and freshly ground
   black pepper
5 slider buns, small French bread rolls,
   or dinner rolls
⅔ cup baby spinach
1 tomato, sliced

1. Combine the chicken, cranberries, pecans, bell pepper, shallot, mustard, yogurt, and salt and black pepper to taste in a medium bowl and mix well.

2. Slice the buns horizontally into thirds (removing the middle third of the bun as described in the headnote). Layer the spinach on the bottom half of each bun and top with tomato. Use an ice cream scoop or spoon to dollop the chicken salad onto each tomato slice. Top with the top third of each bun and squish down a little to secure the sliders.

NOTE: Go ahead and eat two if you're super hungry—two sliders are just 302 calories!

This recipe is a great use for leftover chicken, but if you don't have any available leftovers, just coat a chicken breast with ½ teaspoon olive oil and a little salt and pepper. Place in a skillet over medium-high heat, cover, and cook for 4 to 6 minutes per side, until it feels firm and is cooked through (no pink on the inside).

If you prefer shredded chicken, or find the chopping too time-consuming, shred the chicken with two forks.

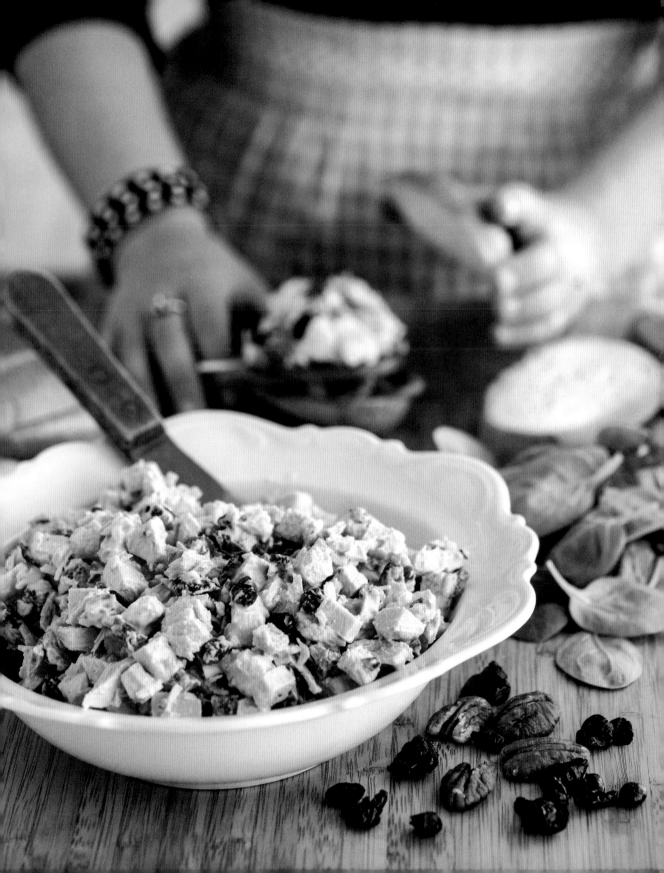

Roast Beef Sandwich with Creamy Horseradish Spread

Makes 4 sandwiches
Serving size: 1 sandwich
Per serving: calories 272; fat 8 g; fiber 3 g; protein 25.5 g; carbohydrates 24 g

A popular chain bakery makes a delicious roast beef sandwich, but it's almost 800 calories! Sure, I could split it with someone, or I could give the sandwich a makeover, cut the calories, and have an even bigger sandwich all to myself. Guess what I chose to do?

My husband loves this recipe. I make it for lunches, picnics, and even some dinners! Get the meat from the deli counter and bread from the bakery section of your grocery store. You want the best for these ingredients, as they carry the weight of the recipe. I also use leftover steak when I have it—if you have extra "Everything" Rubbed Steak (page 168), this is a great way to use it up. The super-skinny horseradish spread adds loads of flavor and virtually no calories. If you like it spicy, go ahead and double up on the horseradish spread, or leave a small bowl of it and a little spoon on the table for everyone to add as much as he or she likes.

Supersize option: Double up the veggies!

Creamy Horseradish Spread
¼ cup 0% Greek yogurt
1 tablespoon freshly grated horseradish (ask your produce manager where to find it; see Note)

Sandwiches
4 whole wheat sandwich rolls
4 teaspoons shredded Asiago cheese (Parmesan or cheddar also works)
4 to 8 romaine lettuce leaves
1 tomato, cut into 8 slices
¼ red onion, thinly sliced
16 slices roast beef or thinly sliced leftover steak
4 slices low-fat cheddar cheese

1. Make the creamy horseradish spread: Combine the yogurt and horseradish in a small bowl and set aside.

2. Make the sandwiches: Preheat the broiler to low or 350°F. If you can't set your broiler to low or a temperature, just heat it up and watch the rolls closely so they don't burn.

3. Place the rolls on a baking sheet and sprinkle the top of each one with 1 teaspoon of the Asiago cheese. Broil for 3 to 5 minutes, until the cheese melts and starts to brown, but watch closely so the rolls don't burn. Remove from the oven and let the cheese set, about 5 minutes.

4. Slice the rolls in half, smear the bottom halves with creamy horseradish sauce, and layer on the lettuce, tomato, red onion, beef, cheese, and more sauce, if you like.

5. Cut the sandwiches in half and serve.

NOTE: Some varieties of jarred horseradish are packed full of preservatives that can cause fat storage and weight gain, so look for the raw. But if you can't find raw horseradish and have to buy jarred, look for organic or refrigerated brands, don't buy anything with the word *creamy* on the label, and *read the ingredients*.

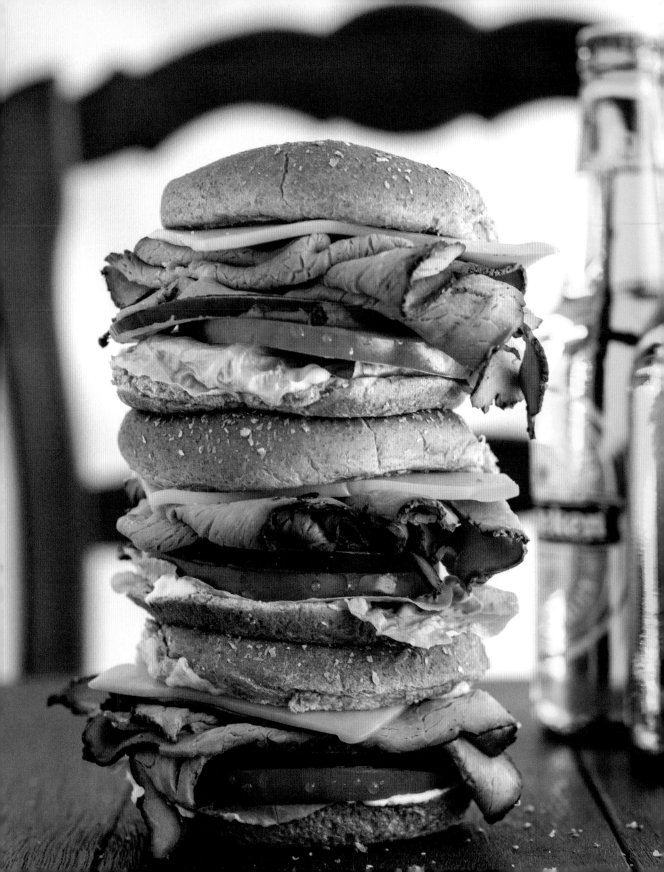

Sausage and Pepper Hoagie

Makes 4 hoagies
Serving size: 1 hoagie
Per serving: calories 224; fat 7.5 g; fiber 4.5 g; protein 14 g; carbohydrates 27 g

Yum, sausage and peppers! I make this with pasta and to top bread as bruschetta and, of course, in these hoagies. This is a great, fast weeknight meal that kids and adults both adore. I swap out the typical fatty sausages for lean turkey sausages, double the veggies, and hollow out the rolls to lose some calories and carbs.

1 teaspoon olive oil
2 organic Italian turkey sausages
1 red bell pepper, roughly chopped
1 green bell pepper, roughly chopped
1 white onion, roughly chopped
2 cloves garlic, chopped
2 tablespoons Italian seasoning
Kosher salt and freshly ground
    black pepper
4 whole wheat hoagie rolls

1. In a large sauté pan, heat the olive oil over medium heat. Add the sausages and brown on all sides, about 10 minutes.

2. Add the bell peppers, onion, garlic, Italian seasoning, and salt and pepper to taste. Cook, stirring often, until the sausages are nearly done, about 10 minutes.

3. Remove the sausages and slice them in half lengthwise. Return them to the pan, cut-side down, along with any juices, to brown and finish cooking, 3 to 5 minutes.

4. Meanwhile, hollow out the center of each roll. Use your fingers to scrape out about a third of the bread on the inside and transfer to a freezer bag to save for homemade bread crumbs (see page 81).

5. Place a sausage half on each roll and top with lots of veggies. Scoop any leftover sauce out of the pan and drizzle it over the filling. If you're feeling ladylike, slice in half, and enjoy!

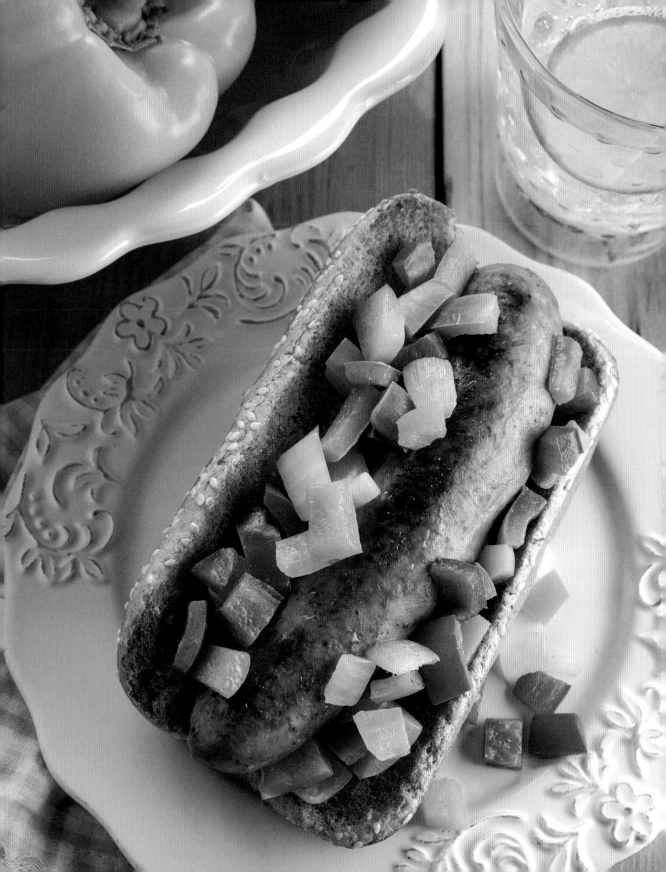

Meatball Sliders

Makes 10 sliders
Serving size: 1 slider
Per serving: calories 207; fat 7 g; fiber 2 g; protein 15 g; carbohydrates 21.5 g

I don't want to live in a world without meatball sandwiches! Of course this typically high-calorie, high-fat, and low-nutrition dish required a little nip and tuck. I added hidden veggies and swapped in turkey for beef to cut the fat and calories. These sliders are the perfect party finger food, family- and kid-friendly main dish, or potluck staple. Serve with a crisp salad or Red and Green Brussels Sprouts (page 228).

1 teaspoon olive oil
1 onion, finely chopped
1 clove garlic, chopped
1 red bell pepper, finely chopped
1 tablespoon Italian seasoning
⅛ teaspoon kosher salt
1 (28-ounce) can organic tomato sauce
1 pound lean ground turkey
1 large egg
2 tablespoons freshly grated Parmesan cheese, plus 3 tablespoons shredded Parmesan cheese
2 tablespoons bread crumbs (see Note)
¼ teaspoon freshly ground black pepper
10 small French rolls or slider buns
3 cups baby spinach

1. In a large sauté pan, heat the oil over medium-high heat. Add the onion, garlic, bell pepper, Italian seasoning, and salt. Cook until the vegetables are soft, about 10 minutes, then transfer to a large bowl to cool.

2. Add the tomato sauce to the pan and reduce the heat to low.

3. Preheat the oven to 350°F.

4. When the vegetables are cool, add the turkey, egg, grated Parmesan cheese, bread crumbs, and pepper to the bowl. Mix until just combined. Do not overmix—it will make tough meatballs.

5. Roll the mixture into ten meatballs about the size of Ping-Pong balls and gently set them in the hot tomato sauce, spooning a little sauce over them as you work. When all the meatballs are in the pan, spoon more sauce over them and cover the pan. Increase the heat to medium and cook the meatballs, turning them and covering them with more sauce as they cook, for 20 minutes.

6. Meanwhile, place the rolls on a baking sheet and sprinkle them with the shredded Parmesan cheese. Bake for 5 to 8 minutes, or until the cheese has melted. Set the rolls aside to cool.

7. Slice the buns horizontally into thirds, cutting off the top and bottom and leaving a slice of bread in the middle. Freeze the middle slices to make croutons (see page 72) or bread crumbs (see Note, opposite).

8. Place the bun bottoms on a platter or individual plates and top each with spinach. (The spinach will wilt and reduce significantly when you add the hot meatballs, so don't be shy.) Top each with a hot meatball, a dollop of sauce, and a crispy cheese bun top and serve.

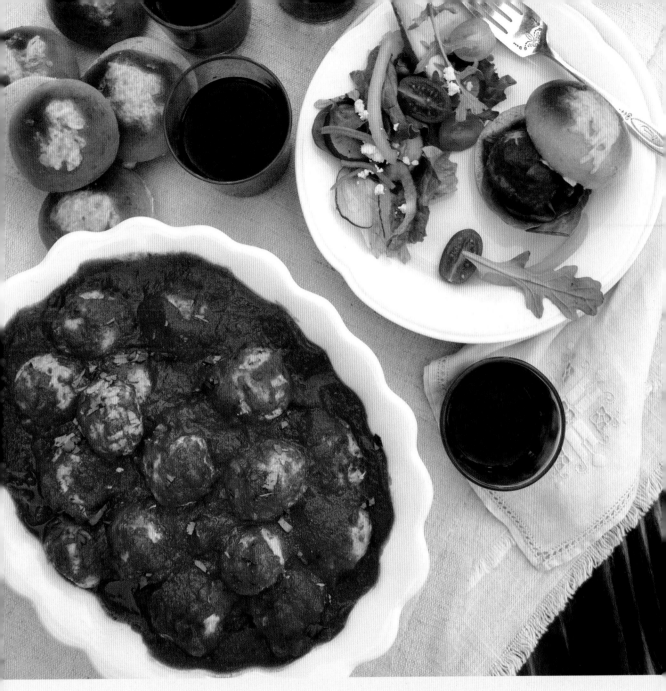

NOTE: You can make the meatballs in a slow cooker if you like; cook on High for 3 hours or on Low for 6 hours.

To make homemade bread crumbs, simply grind one or more slices of bread into crumbs in a food processor. Add ¼ teaspoon Italian seasoning per slice of bread for Italian-style bread crumbs. For crunchier bread crumbs, spread them out on a rimmed cookie sheet and toast in the oven at 350°F for 5 to 10 minutes, until the desired brownness is reached.

Skinny Sloppy Joes

Makes 6 sandwiches
Serving size: 1 sandwich
Per serving: calories 246; fat 9.5 g; fiber 8.5 g; protein 27 g; carbohydrates 54 g

These sloppy joes are the ultimate hidden veggie meal. My husband detests carrots, and I take this as a challenge. The French have an attitude about food and picky eaters: if you don't like it, then you just haven't tried it enough times. That's how I approach food my family doesn't like. In this dish, I grate the carrots and they just blend in with the sauce and meat, helping to sweeten the dish without extra sugar. I also add red bell pepper. If you're dealing with picky eaters, be sure to use red or orange peppers or you'll lose the benefit of stealth.

My mother-in-law makes a knock-your-socks-off sloppy joe, so I asked her to send me her recipe. It was a very old-fashioned recipe that her mother used to make on their family farm in Michigan. I did my best to give homage to this amazing recipe, and even my husband said it was spot on. Try it yourself—it's more than 50 percent veggies and almost as easy as opening up a can of the store-bought stuff.

1 teaspoon olive oil
1 onion, finely chopped
1 red bell pepper, finely chopped
3 cloves garlic, finely chopped
⅛ teaspoon salt
1 pound lean ground turkey
1 carrot, grated
1 (6-ounce) can organic tomato paste
1 (16-ounce) can organic tomato sauce
1 tablespoon Dijon mustard
1 tablespoon pure maple syrup
1 tablespoon balsamic vinegar
1 teaspoon chili powder
1 tablespoon paprika
Freshly ground black pepper
6 whole wheat buns

1. In a large sauté pan, heat the oil over medium heat. Add the onion, bell pepper, garlic, and salt and sauté until the onion is transparent, about 10 minutes. Add the ground turkey and cook, stirring occasionally, until the turkey is browned, about 10 minutes.

2. Add the carrot, tomato paste, tomato sauce, mustard, maple syrup, balsamic vinegar, chili powder, paprika, and black pepper to taste and stir. Simmer until thickened, about 10 minutes.

3. Serve on whole wheat buns.

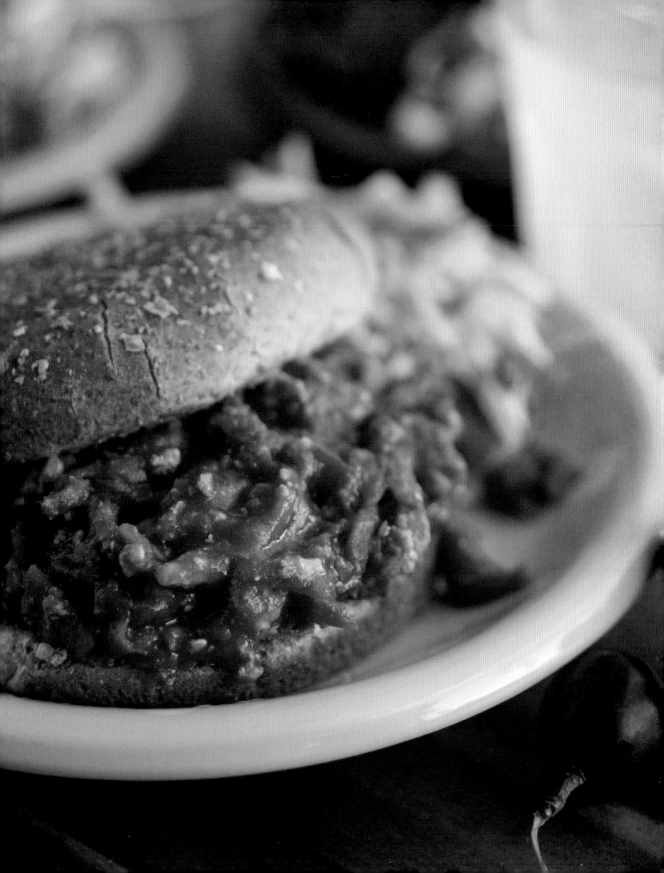

California Muffuletta

Makes 2 sandwiches
Serving size: 1 sandwich
Per serving: calories 322; fat 4.5 g; fiber 4 g; protein 11 g; carbohydrates 48.5 g

This yummy sandwich embodies both the veggie-loving California coast and the heart of New Orleans, the two places I lived in my childhood years. This is not what you might expect from a veggie sandwich: it's huge—not at all wimpy—and so filling you may find yourself unable to finish it!

I often get the same question: "What detox do you recommend?" My answer is always "Lots and lots of veggies and as much water as you can drink." This is a great example of lots and lots of veggies, and best of all, the bread's filling fiber means you won't find yourself with carbohydrate cravings in the afternoon.

8 Kalamata olives
¼ teaspoon juice from the olive jar, plus more as needed
2 ciabatta bread rolls (whole wheat if you can find them), halved
2 slices low-fat sharp cheddar cheese
½ avocado, thinly sliced
½ cup arugula
½ cucumber, cut into 8 thin slices
1 red bell pepper
¼ red onion, cut into 4 slices

1. In a blender or small food processor, combine the olives and olive juice and blend until only small chunks remain. Add a little more olive juice if needed to make a smooth mixture. Spread the olive mixture over the top halves of the rolls and top with the cheese.

2. Lay the avocado on the bottom halves of the rolls and top with the arugula and cucumber.

3. Cut the bell pepper into quarters, remove the seeds and ribs, and press down with the palm of your hand until the pepper cracks and flattens. Divide the bell pepper and onion slices between the bottom halves of the sandwiches.

4. Carefully put the sandwiches together and slice them in half. Don't worry if some veggies spill out—this dish is meant to be messy!

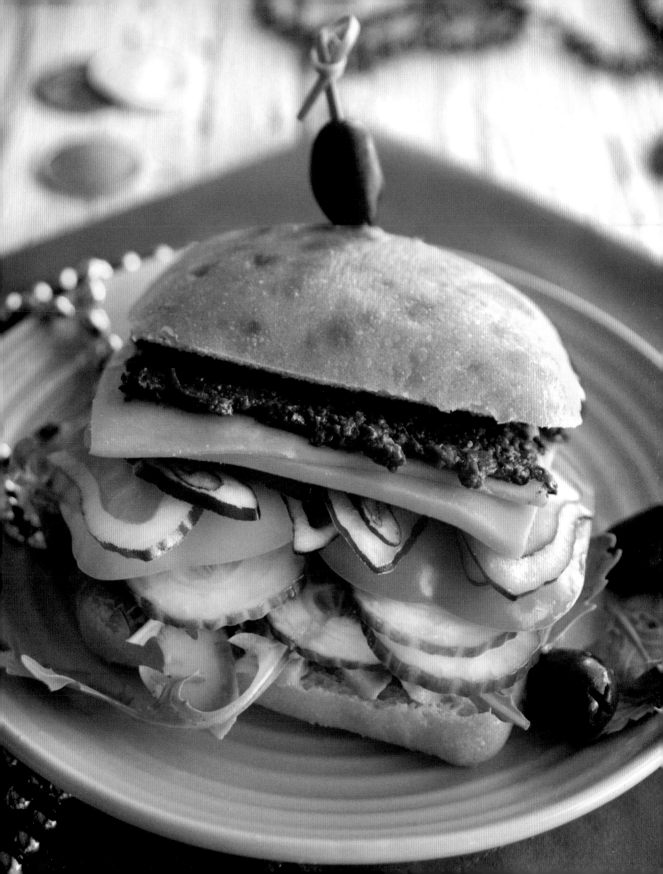

Pesto Chicken Sandwich

Makes 2 sandwiches
Serving size: 1 sandwich
Per serving: calories 442; fat 3 g; fiber 4 g; protein 58 g; carbohydrates 56 g

I'm a little addicted to these sandwiches. For a two-month span, I ate them four days a week for lunch! They're so flavorful and hearty that I'll cut one in half and save the rest for later. If you tend to snack in the late afternoon, just have the second half of the sandwich. You won't be eating any extra calories—you'll just be spreading them out! This works for breakfast and dinner, too, so think about when you tend to snack and plan accordingly.

These sandwiches work great for picnics. I live in wine country, and I make these often when my friends come to visit. We enjoy a glass of chardonnay in the vineyards with a sandwich, which I put on sourdough rolls just to make them a little fancier (and a little heartier, which guys love).

1 boneless, skinless chicken breast
1 teaspoon olive oil
Kosher salt and freshly ground
    black pepper
4 slices whole wheat sourdough bread
¼ cup shredded sharp cheddar cheese
¼ cup 0% Greek yogurt
1 tablespoon Skinny Pesto (page 71)
½ avocado, sliced
½ cup arugula

1. Brush the chicken with the olive oil and sprinkle it with salt and pepper. In a large sauté or grill pan, cook the chicken over medium heat for 5 minutes on each side, or until there is no pink in the center. Set the chicken aside for 5 minutes to cool, then thinly slice it.

2. Preheat the broiler.

3. Lightly toast the bread in a toaster. Lay 2 slices of toast on a baking sheet and top them with the cheese. Broil for 1 to 3 minutes, until the cheese starts to melt. Set aside to cool a little.

4. In a small bowl, combine the Greek yogurt and pesto. Spread it over the slices of toast without cheese. Top with the chicken, avocado, and arugula.

5. Put the sandwiches together and press them gently. Cut in half and enjoy.

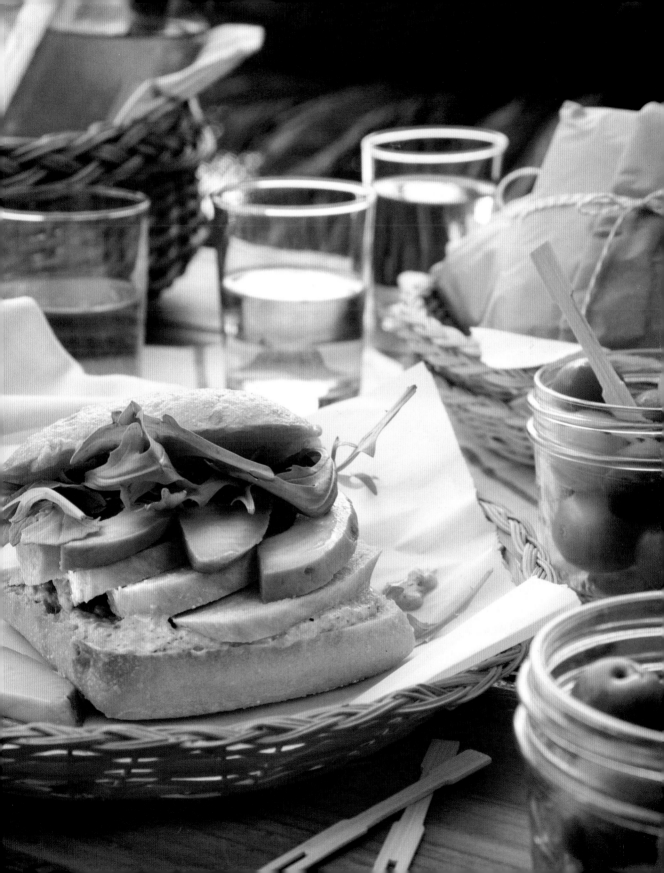

Chapter 5

Cheese Wiz

Life is far too short to give up mac and cheese and nachos, but don't fret—these naughty delights can be made with half the calories of the originals, so you can feel good about making cheesy dishes for the family or just yourself.

My favorite Smart Swaps for this chapter:

Almond milk is only 60 calories per cup—half the calories of 2% milk and just as creamy.

Greek yogurt has only one-third the calories of light sour cream and almost exactly the same flavor.

Sharp cheese: The sharper the better! Sharp cheese has more flavor than mild, so you don't need as much to get all the yummy cheesy flavor.

Creamy Mac and Cheese

Makes 6 servings
Serving size: ½ cup
Per serving: calories 312; fat 8 g; fiber 7.5 g; protein 11 g; carbohydrates 50 g

---

My daughter and I love mac and cheese. It's a great side dish with dinner and a great lunch served with a crisp salad! I never make it the same way twice. I'm always adding toppings, hidden veggies, and even leftover roasted chicken or turkey when it's handy. This recipe is the base. Try it yourself and check out the toppings and add-ins I've provided on the opposite page, and don't be shy—pull out your pen and make some notes on your favorite toppings!

An important tip: Use sharp cheese, the sharper the better. You'll get the same rich, cheesy flavor with fewer calories and less fat.

1 (13.25-ounce) box whole wheat elbow
   pasta
1 tablespoon unsalted butter
1 tablespoon all-purpose flour
3 cups unsweetened almond milk
½ cup grated sharp cheddar cheese

1. Bring a large saucepan of water to a boil. Add the pasta and cook until al dente according to the package directions. Drain and set aside.

2. In the same pan, melt the butter over medium-low heat. Add the flour and mix with a wooden spoon, stirring continuously for about 5 minutes, or until you have a lightly browned paste (this is the roux).

3. Add 1 cup of the almond milk and whisk well, breaking up any lumps. Stir in the remaining 2 cups almond milk and increase the heat to medium-high. Cook, stirring continuously and occasionally scraping the bottom of the pan with the wooden spoon, until the mixture has thickened and coats the spoon with little to no transparency. Turn off the heat.

4. Stir in the pasta until it's covered in the sauce. Add the cheese and mix until it has melted and is evenly distributed.

5. Serve with a crunchy green salad (see my Guide to the Perfect Salad, page 18).

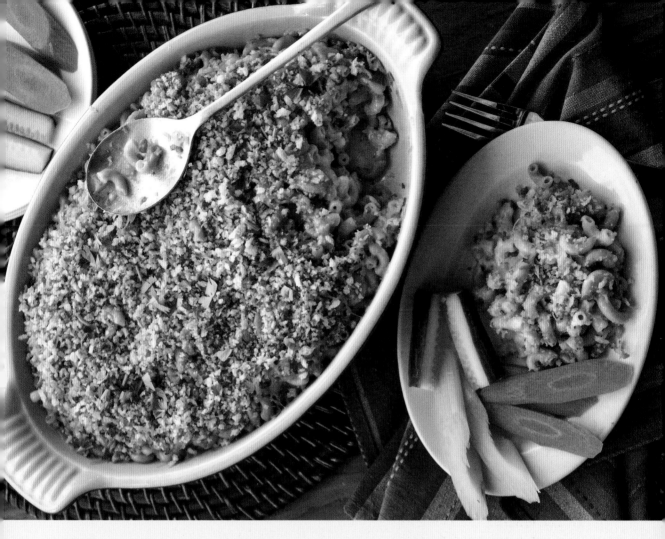

Truffle Mac and Cheese: Use truffle butter or truffle oil instead of butter and sprinkle 1 tablespoon truffle salt in with the cheese.

Bacon Jalapeño: Cook 1 slice bacon in the pan and use 1 tablespoon of the drippings in place of the butter. Crumble the bacon and set aside. Seed and chop 2 jalapeños and add half the jalapeños with the cheese. Sprinkle the top of the mac and cheese with the remaining jalapeños and the crumbled bacon.

Crunchy Top: Transfer the mac and cheese to a baking dish and sprinkle the top with ¼ cup panko bread crumbs and 2 tablespoons grated Parmesan cheese. Broil for 2 to 5 minutes, or until golden brown and crispy. Watch carefully, or it may burn!

Hidden Veggies: Add your desired combination of ½ cup cubed cooked chicken, ¼ cup frozen corn, ½ cup diced cauliflower, and ¼ cup diced butternut squash (chop the veggies the same size or smaller than the cooked pasta). Toss the cauliflower and butternut squash in 1 teaspoon olive oil on a baking sheet and roast at 350°F for 35 minutes. Add the chicken, corn, and cooked veggies to the pasta with the cheese.

Twice-Baked Cheesy Potato Boats

Makes 6 potato boats
Serving size: 1 potato boat
Per serving: calories 116; fat 1.5 g; fiber 1.5 g; protein 6 g; carbohydrates 20.5 g

The individual portions make these ideal for parties and holiday gatherings, but these potato boats are so easy that you'll find yourself whipping them up on weeknights.

Greek yogurt is the secret weapon in this recipe. It holds the potato boats together and adds creaminess and protein. Even if you don't like Greek yogurt, try it in this recipe. You won't taste it, but you'll benefit from its metabolism-boosting qualities and might just find a new way to love a healthy ingredient.

3 medium russet potatoes
2 green onions, thinly sliced
¼ cup small-cubed sharp cheddar cheese
¾ cup 0% Greek yogurt
1½ tablespoons Five-Minute Salsa
  (page 96) or your favorite salsa
  or hot sauce
½ teaspoon kosher salt
½ teaspoon freshly ground black pepper

1. Preheat the oven to 350°F.

2. Scrub the potatoes in cool water and pierce them a few times with a fork. Bake the potatoes for 1 hour, or until soft in the center. (If you're in a rush, microwave the fork-pierced potatoes for 10 to 15 minutes.)

3. In a large bowl, combine the onions, cheese, yogurt, salsa or hot sauce, salt, and pepper.

4. Slice the potatoes in half lengthwise. Scoop out the potato flesh into the bowl, leaving a small layer around the sides and on the bottom so the potato skins hold together. Set the potato skin "boats" on a rimmed baking sheet.

5. Mix the potato mixture well with a fork, mashing the potato as you go.

6. Divide the potato mixture evenly among the potato boats and bake for 15 minutes, or until the cheese starts to melt and the center is piping hot. (If you're taking them to a party or holiday gathering, you can assemble the boats, cover the baking sheet with aluminum foil, and do the baking at your destination.)

For a kid-friendly dish, use organic ketchup instead of salsa or hot sauce.

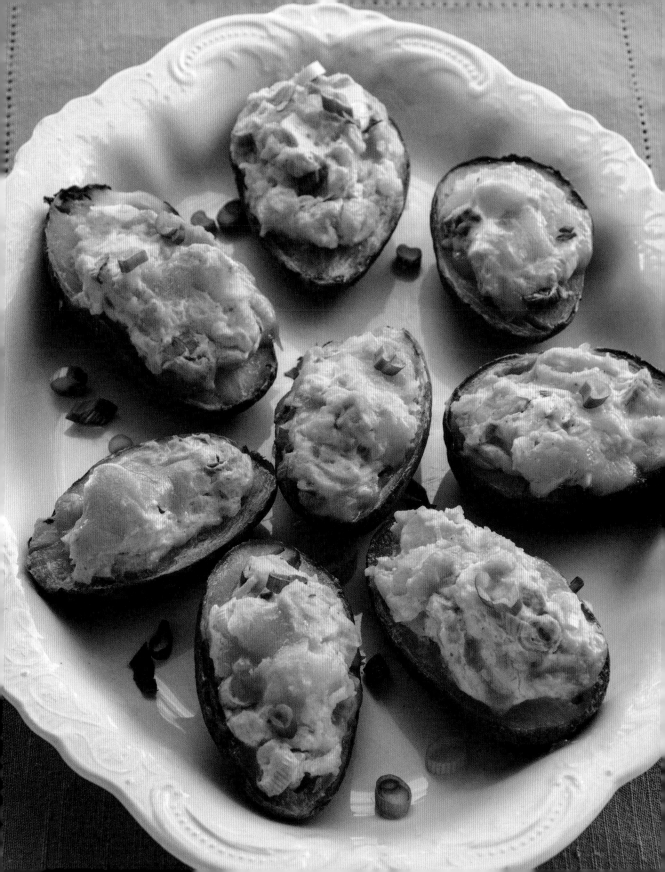

Chicken, Avocado, and Cheddar Quesadilla

Makes 4 quesadillas
Serving size: 1 quesadilla
Per serving: calories 307; fat 16.5 g; fiber 5.5 g; protein 14.5 g; carbohydrates 26 g

---

These cheesy quesadillas are delicious and easy to make. I top each one with a big dollop of Greek yogurt in place of sour cream and serve them with Black Bean Avocado Salad (page 192).

If you have leftover chicken, use it in these! I find it's easy to keep my grocery bill low by using my leftovers wisely, so instead of leaving your leftovers in the fridge where you and your family are more likely to snack, freeze them in individual or family serving sizes for fast weeknight meals.

1 teaspoon olive oil
1 boneless, skinless chicken breast
4 whole wheat tortillas
½ cup grated sharp cheddar cheese
1 avocado, sliced
0% Greek yogurt (optional)

1. In a large skillet, heat the oil over medium heat. Add the chicken and cook for 5 minutes per side, until cooked through with no pink in the middle. Turn off the heat and transfer the chicken to a plate until cool enough to handle. Reserve the drippings in the pan.

2. Shred the chicken into small bites. Reheat the pan over medium heat.

3. Lay the tortillas out on a clean surface. Over half of each tortilla, spread 1 tablespoon of the cheese. Divide the avocado slices, shredded chicken, and remaining cheese among the tortillas. Fold each tortilla into a half-moon and place the quesadillas in the hot skillet. Cook for 5 to 8 minutes on each side, or until the tortillas are lightly browned and the cheese has melted.

4. Move the quesadillas to a cutting board and use scissors or a pizza wheel to slice each into four triangles. Top with Greek yogurt, if desired, and serve.

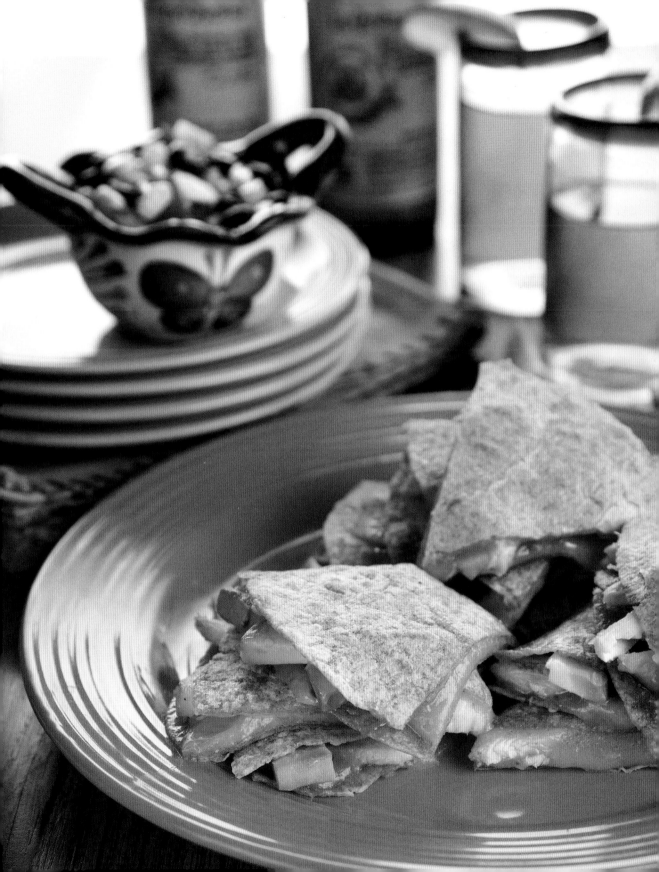

Game-Day Nacho Dip

Makes 20 servings
Serving size: ¼ cup
Per serving: calories 129; fat 3 g; fiber 5 g; protein 12 g; carbohydrates 14 g

My nachos have long been a family favorite, but to be frank, they don't travel well. I came up with this travel-friendly nacho dip when someone requested it for a potluck. It's now a personal favorite because it's easier to make than the original! I bring this to almost every party I attend, and it's a hit among all the men at Super Bowl parties. They have no clue that I've swapped in Greek yogurt for sour cream . . . until now.

I serve this dip with my Easy Tortilla Chips (page 116) and veggie sticks. I highly recommend that you make it in a clear bowl to show off its colorful layers.

1 teaspoon olive oil
1 white or yellow onion, chopped
1 red bell pepper, chopped
1 clove garlic, chopped
⅛ teaspoon salt
1 pound lean ground turkey
1 teaspoon chili powder
1 tablespoon dried oregano
2 cups 0% Greek yogurt

2 (15-ounce) cans low-sodium black beans, drained and rinsed
1 cup shredded low-fat sharp cheddar cheese
2 cups Guacamole Dip (page 104)
2 cups Five-Minute Salsa (below) or your favorite salsa
1 jalapeño, sliced into rings (optional)

1. In a large sauté pan, heat the olive oil over medium-high heat. Add the onion, bell pepper, garlic, and salt and cook until the veggies are soft, about 10 minutes.

2. Add the turkey, chili powder, and oregano and cook, stirring occasionally, for 15 minutes, or until the turkey is cooked through. Set aside to cool to room temperature.

3. Spread the turkey mixture on the bottom of a large, deep glass bowl, followed by the Greek yogurt. Layer the black beans over the Greek yogurt and sprinkle the cheese over the beans. Spoon the guacamole over the cheese and spread it out in an even layer. Pour the salsa over the guacamole and smooth the top. Garnish with jalapeño rings, if desired.

Five-Minute Salsa

5 large tomatoes, chopped
1 red onion, chopped
3 jalapeños, seeded and chopped
¼ cup fresh cilantro, chopped
Juice of 1 lime
Kosher salt and freshly ground black pepper

1. Toss the tomatoes, onion, jalapeños, and cilantro in a medium bowl. Add the lime juice and salt and pepper to taste. Refrigerate the salsa overnight for maximum flavor. It will keep in the fridge for up to 4 days.

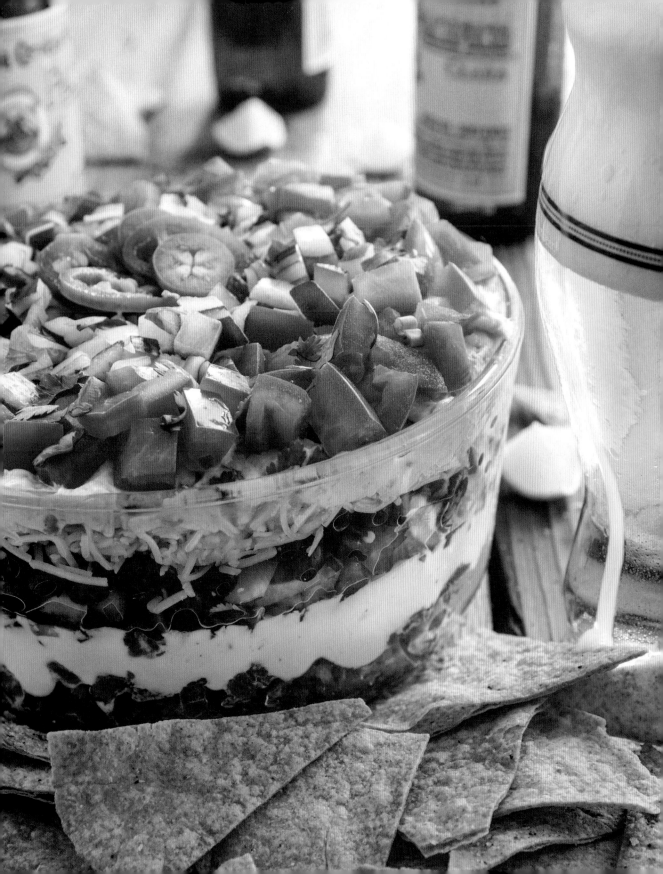

Mini Cheesy Pretzel Dogs

Makes 24 pretzel dogs
Serving size: 1 pretzel dog
Per serving: calories 36; fat 1.5 g; fiber 0 g; protein 1 g; carbohydrates 4 g

---

These have become so popular on my blog that I had to include them in this book, but I did give them a little makeover while I was at it, adding flavor and even dropping a few calories! Be sure to grate a good-quality sharp cheese as fine as you can—this way you get more flavor for your calories.

Regular hot dogs are basically mystery meat full of chemicals like nitrates and preservatives. These nasty chemicals not only won't help your weight loss, but they'll add weight and slowly make you sick. Make sure you get organic, nitrate-free chicken hot dogs. You can't tell the difference in this recipe, and the cost difference is only about a dollar per pack.

These are great for parties and kids' sleepovers, and at only 36 calories each you can have six of them for only 216 calories. Serve with a salad or Ranch Dip (page 105) with veggie sticks for a kid-friendly dinner, and freeze your leftovers for fast weeknight dinners—they can be stored in the freezer for up to 4 months!

Pretzel Dogs

1 cup self-rising flour, plus more as needed
½ teaspoon kosher salt
1 teaspoon garlic powder
3 tablespoons grated sharp cheese
    (I like a combo of cheddar, Parmesan, and pepper Jack)
½ cup unsweetened almond milk
1½ tablespoons olive oil
1 large egg, beaten
8 nitrate-free organic chicken hot dogs, cut crosswise into thirds

Egg Wash

1 egg white
¼ teaspoon kosher salt

1. Preheat the oven to 425°F. Line two baking sheets with parchment paper.

2. In the bowl of a stand mixer fitted with the dough hook or in a large bowl, mix the flour, salt, garlic powder, and cheese.

3. In a medium bowl, whisk together the almond milk, oil, and egg.

4. Add the wet ingredients to the dry ingredients and mix until just combined. You may need to add a little more flour as you mix; you want the dough to be slightly sticky, but not so sticky that you can't roll it out.

5. Transfer half the dough to a clean, flour-dusted surface. Dust a rolling pin with flour and roll out the dough into a 12-inch square. Slice with a pizza wheel horizontally down the middle once and vertically six times to make twelve rectangles of dough.

6. Roll a piece of dough around each mini dog (some of the hot dog ends will poke out, which is okay) and place them on the prepared baking sheet as you go. Roll out the remaining dough to wrap the rest of the mini dogs.

7. In a small bowl, beat the egg white with the salt and 1 teaspoon water to make an egg wash. Brush the tops of the dough lightly with the egg wash. Bake the pretzel dogs for 12 to 15 minutes, or until the dough is golden brown.

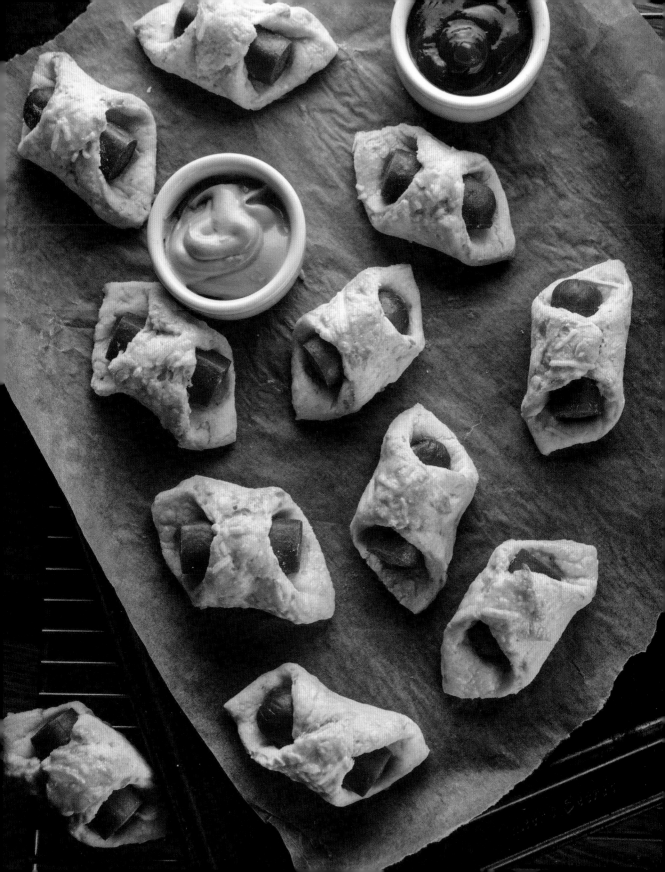

· Chapter 6 ·

Snack Lovers

When people say eating healthy is too expensive, it's usually the snacks that are driving up their grocery budget. Premade snacks from the store are full of artificial sweeteners and colors, fat-storing preservatives, and other chemicals, and they cost a small fortune.

Stop spending money on food that's making you unhealthy and slowing down your weight loss, and start making your own! Be sure to check out the twenty-five snacks under 100 calories in this chapter for less expensive and more filling, more nutritious, and far more delicious snacks than the 100-calorie packs you find at the store.

My favorite Smart Swaps for this chapter:

Greek yogurt is one of my favorite dip ingredients. I use it in place of sour cream and even whipped cream to cut calories and boost protein content.

Unsweetened applesauce can be used in place of butter and sugar when baking.

Veggie sticks are a healthier option when it comes to snacking—they have all the crunch of chips for a fraction of the calories.

Four Metabolism-Boosting
Greek Yogurt Dips with Veggie Sticks

I wanted to include some lunch box snacks— and I'm talking about your lunch box, not your kid's. The following dips are perfect for eating at your desk or, better yet, outside at a picnic bench in the sunlight.

If you usually make dips with sour cream, you'll be pleasantly surprised at how close in flavor and consistency Greek yogurt is. It's significantly lower in calories and fat and naturally boosts your metabolism—just make sure you get 0% and unsweetened.

I love these dips with crunchy vegetables. It's a great way to give your body what it needs and turn off your hunger receptors. You'll find you stay full longer and feel much more satisfied. Here are some veggies that go great with the dips that follow. They boost metabolism and give you that crunch you crave in chips and crackers.

Speaking of chips and crackers, I do have some all-natural options, such as Easy Tortilla Chips (page 116), BBQ-Flavored Potato Chips (page 113), and Rosemary Olive Oil Wheat Crackers (page 118), but you'll find you can have much more food if you opt for all or at least half veggies. Choose among these:

Bell pepper sticks

Carrot sticks

Celery stalks

Cucumber slices

Endive leaves

Fennel slices

Jicama sticks

Radish slices

Zucchini slices

To store these dips for later, cut a slice of plastic wrap larger than the container you're using, press it directly against the surface of the dip, and press down to remove any air bubbles. Cover the container with its lid and refrigerate the dip for up to 3 days. Stir before serving.

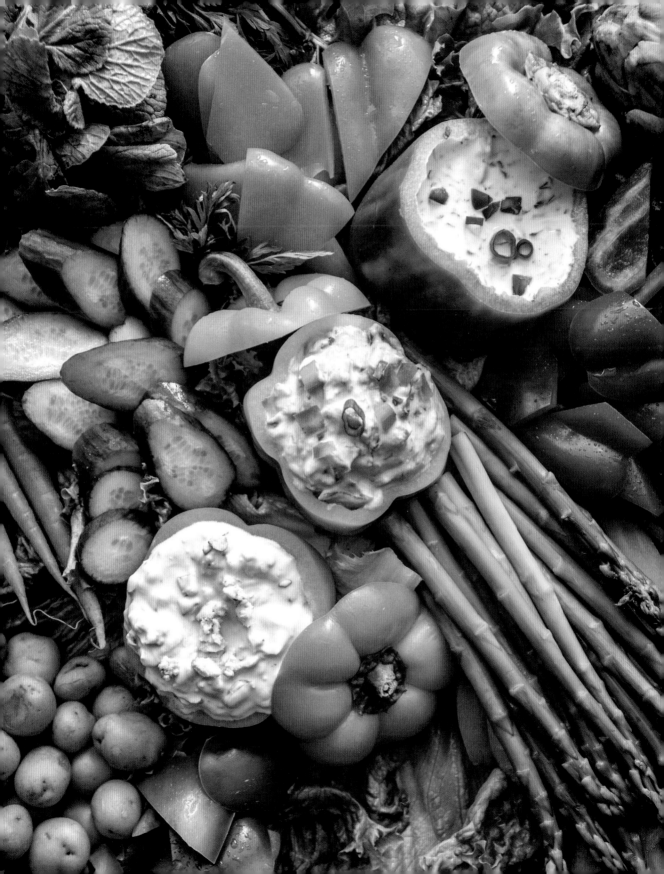

Guacamole Dip

Makes 4 servings
Serving size: ⅓ cup
Per serving: calories 108; fat 7 g; fiber 2 g; protein 5 g; carbohydrates 5 g

---

This guacamole had to be the first dip recipe featured—it's my personal favorite. Avocados are a superfood, full of good fats that leave your hair shiny and skin glowing. You gotta love a snack that fills you up and makes you pretty!

I use my Five-Minute Salsa in this recipe, and once in a while I use my favorite hot sauce instead. If you have a favorite salsa or hot sauce that's all natural, by all means use it here— recipes are meant to be flexible.

1 avocado
½ clove garlic
⅔ cup 0% Greek yogurt
4 to 6 tablespoons Five-Minute Salsa
   (page 96)
Juice of ½ lime
1 tomato, seeded and diced
1 green onion, chopped
1 jalapeño, seeded and minced
Kosher salt and freshly ground
   black pepper
Veggie sticks (see page 102), for serving

1. Cut the avocado in half, remove the pit, and scoop the flesh out into a medium bowl. Use a fine grater to shred the garlic clove into the bowl. If you want the guacamole super spicy, add more garlic.

2. Smash the avocado and garlic together with the back of a fork until smooth. Add the yogurt, salsa, lime juice, tomato, onion, jalapeño, and a pinch of salt and pepper. Mix together, taste, and add more lime juice or salt as needed.

3. Serve with veggie sticks. I love carrots and bell peppers with this one, but you can find more options on page 102.

Ranch Dip

Makes 4 cups
Serving size: ½ cup
Per serving: calories 28; fat 0 g; fiber 0 g; protein 5 g; carbohydrates 2 g

Who doesn't like ranch, right?! I figured, why fight it? Let's just make a healthy version you can enjoy guilt-free instead of eliminating it altogether! Fresh herbs really do make the difference, but you can substitute a smaller amount of dried herbs if you have to.

½ clove garlic, minced
3 tablespoons minced fresh chives
2 tablespoons minced fresh parsley
½ teaspoon minced fresh dill
1 teaspoon kosher salt
1 teaspoon freshly ground black pepper
2 cups 0% Greek yogurt
1 tablespoon white vinegar
Veggie sticks (see page 102), for serving

1. Combine all the ingredients except the veggie sticks in a blender or food processor and blend until smooth. (If you don't have a blender or food processor, just stir everything together in a bowl—the texture will be different but it will still be delicious.)

2. Serve with veggie sticks. I love cucumber, zucchini, and bell pepper with this one, but you can find more options on page 102.

Ranch Salad Dressing: Add ⅔ cup skim or almond milk to thin the dip into a dressing.

Salsa Ranch Dip: Add ¼ cup salsa (such as Five-Minute Salsa, page 96) and 2 tablespoons chopped fresh cilantro.

Tzatziki Dip

Makes 2 cups
Serving size: ½ cup
Per serving: calories 39; fat 0 g; fiber 1 g; protein 5.5 g; carbohydrates 2 g

This Greek-inspired dip is a crowd-pleaser and beyond easy to make—all you need is a cheese grater, knife, and spoon. I love this on top of leftover Greek Pasta Salad (page 152), cold right out of the fridge.

1 (3-inch) piece cucumber
½ clove garlic
1 cup 0% Greek yogurt
2 tablespoons chopped fresh dill
1 tablespoon chopped fresh parsley
½ teaspoon kosher salt
¼ teaspoon freshly ground black pepper
Veggie sticks (see page 102), for serving

1. Use a fine grater to shred the cucumber and garlic into a medium bowl. Add the yogurt, herbs, salt, and pepper and mix together.

2. Serve with veggie sticks. I love cucumber, carrot, and bell pepper with this one, but you can find more options on page 102.

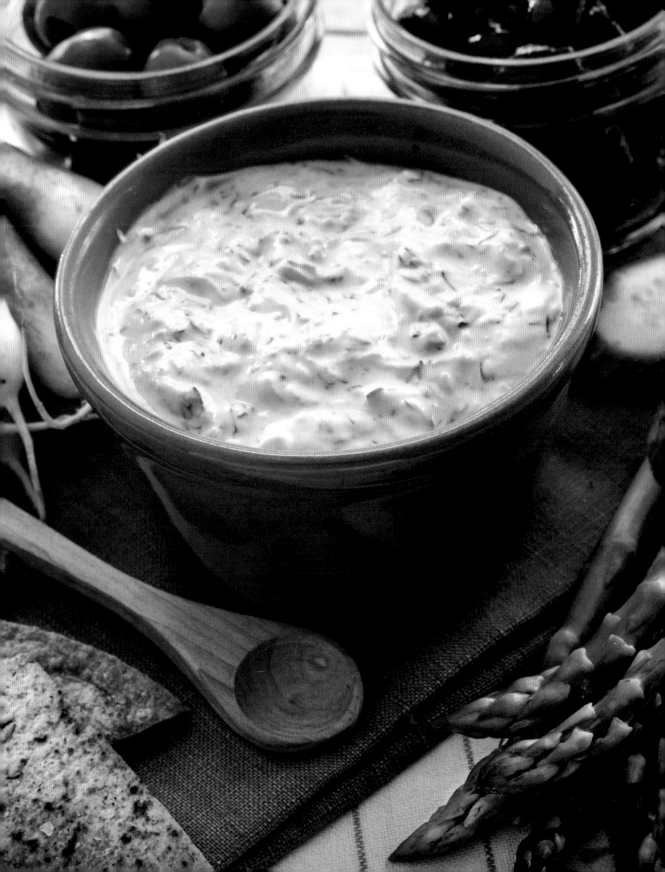

Chunky Blue Cheese Dip

Makes 2 cups
Serving size: ½ cup
Per serving: calories 53; fat 2 g; fiber 0 g; protein 7 g; carbohydrates 2 g

This dip is a family favorite. It's packed with flavor and goes great on burgers or on my Grilled Chicken "Burger" (page 164). I even serve it for dinner with veggie sticks and my Lemony Drumsticks (page 172). Blue cheese has a really strong flavor, so a little goes a long way.

4 green onions, thinly sliced
1 cup 0% Greek yogurt
¼ cup crumbled blue cheese
½ teaspoon freshly ground black pepper
Veggie sticks (see page 102), for serving

1. Place the green onions in a medium bowl, reserving 1 tablespoon for garnish. Add the yogurt, blue cheese, and pepper and fold together carefully. Don't smash the cheese too much—you want the dip to have small, medium, and large chunks. Top with the reserved green onions.

2. Serve with veggie sticks. I love carrots and celery with this one, but you can find more options on page 102.

If you want to make this into a salad dressing, just add ⅓ cup skim milk or unsweetened almond milk to thin it out. Store in a glass jar for easy shaking and keep it in your fridge for up to 1 week.

Trail Mix

Makes 15 servings
Serving size: ¼ cup
Per serving: calories 155; fat 10 g; fiber 5 g; protein 4 g; carbohydrates 14 g

---

A few years ago, General Motors named my Skinny Trail Mix one of the top five trail mixes for road trips. Who knew GM read my blog?! I've revamped that delicious trail mix for this book, so if you loved that one, you'll love this one even more.

This trail mix is great for hiking and camping and for healthy road trip snacks, too, of course. I swapped in some great, low-calorie options for the typical chocolate chips, but if you can't find cacao nibs, just use mini semisweet chocolate chips or mini dark chocolate chips. Be sure to get organic and unsweetened fruit. Otherwise, you're adding unnecessary calories. Some health food stores have nuts, dried fruits, and even the cacao nibs sold loose, so you can purchase just what you need.

1 cup almonds
1 cup pumpkin seeds
½ cup dried banana slices
½ cup dried pineapple, chopped
½ cup dried papaya, chopped
⅛ cup unsweetened coconut flakes
⅛ cup cacao nibs

1. In a large container or gallon freezer bag, combine all the ingredients. I like to leave a ¼-cup measuring cup in the bag for easy serving. You can also divide the trail mix into fifteen smaller containers or bags.

Dark Chocolate Chip Granola Bars

Makes 32 bars
Serving size: 1 bar
Per serving: calories 61; fat 2 g; fiber 1 g; protein 2 g; carbohydrates 10 g

Stop spending money on the preservative-filled store-bought bars when you can make them yourself for half the price! Most granola bar recipes are packed with sugar and butter, making them more like cookies and less like health food. I worked on this recipe, reducing the sugar and butter until I had these perfect 61-calorie bars. In the end 1½ cups of sugar were removed along with 4 tablespoons of butter with the help of my secret Smart Swap weapon . . . applesauce! Try this trick yourself: take a favorite high-calorie recipe and swap half the sugar and butter for applesauce. It's a great Smart Swap that works well in baked sweets.

One last applesauce tip: If you don't have any Homemade Applesauce, get the little cups of unsweetened all-natural applesauce at the store. They are about ½ cup each and are great to keep in the pantry for baking on the fly.

¾ cup all-purpose flour, plus more
    for dusting
½ teaspoon baking soda
¼ teaspoon kosher salt
2 tablespoons unsalted butter,
    at room temperature
½ cup packed light brown sugar
1 large egg
2 teaspoons pure vanilla extract
½ cup Homemade Applesauce (page 112)
2 cups old-fashioned rolled oats
½ cup flaxseeds
⅔ cup dark chocolate chips
½ teaspoon olive oil

1. Preheat the oven to 350°F. Line two rimmed baking sheets with parchment paper.

2. In a small bowl, combine the flour, baking soda, and salt.

3. In a large bowl or the bowl of a stand mixer fitted with the paddle attachment, beat the butter and brown sugar on medium until pale. Add the egg, vanilla, and applesauce and beat on low until combined. Add the flour mixture, oats, flaxseeds, and ⅓ cup of the chocolate chips. Mix until just combined; overmixing will give you a tough dough.

4. Transfer the dough to a clean, floured surface and use floured hands to mold it into a large 2 x 1-foot rectangle about 1 inch thick. Use a pizza wheel or large knife to cut the rectangle into four smaller rectangles, then cut each rectangle into eight bars. Use a spatula to move the bars to the prepared baking sheets, spacing them to allow for spreading.

5. Bake for 10 to 15 minutes, or until the bars are golden brown. Transfer the bars to a wire rack to cool.

6. While the bars cool, place the remaining chocolate chips in a microwave-safe bowl and melt the chocolate on high power in 15-second intervals, stirring after each one. Mix in the olive oil (this keeps the chocolate from hardening). Use a spoon to drizzle chocolate over the granola bars. Store in the fridge for 1 week or in the freezer for up to 4 months.

Try swapping white chocolate chips for half the dark chocolate, mixed in or drizzled over the top.

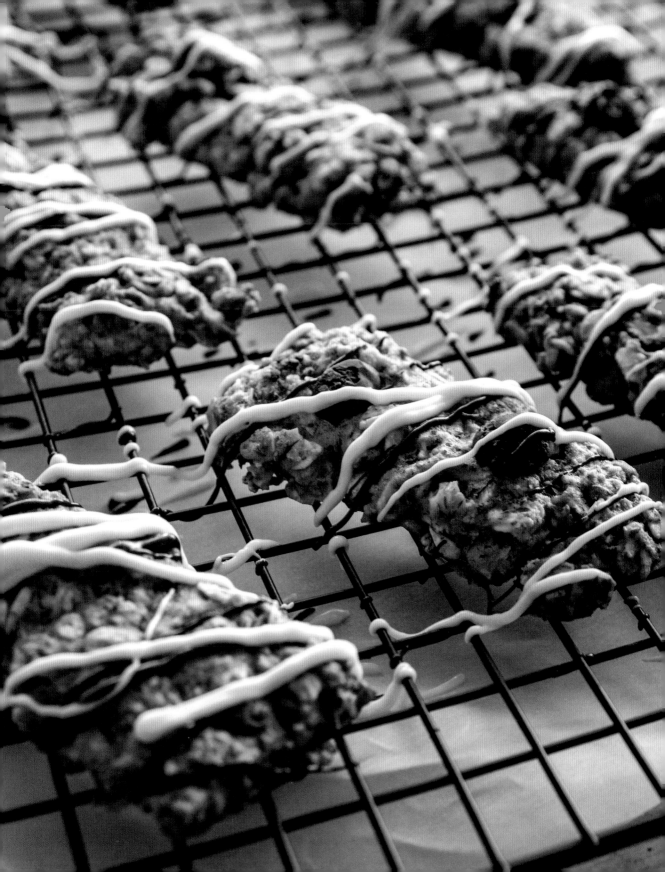

Homemade Applesauce

Serving size: ½ cup
Per serving: calories 137; fat 0 g; fiber 6 g; protein 1 g; carbohydrates 37 g
Makes 5 cups

I love making this easy homemade applesauce. I know exactly what is in it, and I feel comfortable serving it to my family. I serve it as a snack in my daughter's lunch box, but more often I use it in baking recipes to cut out sugar and butter.

You may notice that I cook my applesauce far longer than most recipes call for. By cooking for 45 minutes instead of the usual 25, I can omit all the sugar from the recipe and still come out with a perfectly sweet sauce!

The most tedious part is peeling and slicing the apples. It's not really hard, but it is time-consuming. If you have a peeler/corer/slicer, your job is made easier (you can find one on Amazon.com or WilliamsSonoma.com). If not, do what I do—pop in your favorite movie and set up your cutting board, knife, and saucepan in your living room. Find ways to enjoy your prep work!

1 (6-pound) bag Fuji apples (Honeycrisp
    or Gala work well, too; about 15 large
    apples or 25 small apples)
Juice of 1 orange

1. Peel, core, and thinly slice the apples. Add them to a large saucepan as you work, discarding the skins and cores.

2. Add the orange juice and ⅓ cup water and toss the mixture with a wooden spoon.

3. Cover the pan and place over medium heat. Cook, stirring every 15 minutes, for 45 minutes, or until the apples are soft and sweet. Remove from the heat and let cool for 1 hour (unless you're serving it hot). If you like your applesauce a little chunky, you're done—just let it cool completely before moving to the fridge—but if you are going to use it in baking recipes, be sure to blend as directed in step 4.

4. Transfer the apples and all the liquid to a food processor or blender. (If blending while still hot, remove the little cup on top and cover the open hole with a kitchen towel. Use an oven mitt to protect yourself and place your hand gently over the kitchen towel to hold it in place. This will help avoid pressure buildup. (If you don't do this, opening the lid may result in applesauce spraying all over your kitchen.) Blend until the applesauce is the desired consistency. I like it super smooth, so I blend until there are no chunks, about 3 minutes.

Berry Applesauce: Add 1 cup berries (strawberries, blueberries, raspberries, or all three) to the apples for the last 15 minutes of cooking.

Cinnamon Applesauce: Add 1 teaspoon ground cinnamon and ¼ teaspoon ground nutmeg to the blender.

BBQ-Flavored Potato Chips

Makes about 170 chips
Serving size: 10 chips
Per serving: calories 39; fat 1 g; fiber 1 g; protein 1 g; carbohydrates 6 g

---

I'm not a huge fan of potato chips—they're just too greasy for me—but I do have a soft spot in my heart for BBQ-flavored chips. This delicious BBQ chip recipe can easily be changed into a more traditional potato chip recipe if you like. I won't lie—these can be time-consuming if you have a small single oven—but they're well worth it!

I use a mandoline to slice the potatoes very thin. A mandoline is a very inexpensive and helpful tool in the kitchen. I can't imagine making these without one.

2 large russet potatoes
1 tablespoon olive oil
1½ teaspoons dark brown sugar
1 tablespoon chili powder
1 teaspoon garlic powder
1 teaspoon kosher salt
1 teaspoon freshly ground black pepper

1. Preheat the oven to 375°F. Line three or four rimmed baking sheets with parchment paper.

2. Scrub the potatoes in cold water then slice them very thin using a mandoline. Toss them in a large bowl with the olive oil. Spread the potatoes on the prepared baking sheets, making sure not to overlap them. Bake for 15 to 20 minutes, until brown and crispy.

3. While the potatoes bake, combine the remaining ingredients in a gallon freezer bag. Seal and shake.

4. Remove the chips from the oven and immediately add them to the bag of spices. Seal the bag and shake well to coat all the chips with the seasoning.

5. Transfer the seasoned chips to a plate to cool, and reserve the leftover seasoning for any chips left in the oven. Store the chips in a freezer bag at room temperature for 3 to 4 days.

Original Potato Chips: Omit the seasoning mix and toss the chips with 1 teaspoon kosher salt after removing from the oven.

Chocolate Peanut Butter Dip with Fruit

Makes 2 servings
Serving size: ¼ cup dip and 10 strawberries or 1 apple
Per serving: calories 193; fat 11 g; fiber 4 g; protein 9 g; carbohydrates 18 g
(nutrition information does not include toppings)

This dip takes the traditional apple slices dipped in peanut butter to the next level, and it takes only a minute to make. Kids love it, adults love it—who wouldn't love chocolate peanut butter–dipped strawberries, right?! The Greek yogurt turns this into a fluffy, sweet mousse and helps cut the calories while increasing the protein content.

Get all-natural peanut butter. All that sugar they put in the big-name brands is in no way healthy, and you won't be able to tell the difference in recipes like this one. Almond butter also works well in this, as does any nut butter.

Dip
2 tablespoons all-natural peanut butter
1 tablespoon semisweet chocolate chips
½ cup 0% Greek yogurt

Fruit
20 strawberries, hulled
2 apples, cored and sliced

Toppings (Optional)
2 teaspoons unsweetened flaked coconut
1 tablespoon slivered almonds
2 teaspoons crushed peanuts
2 teaspoons cacao nibs

1. Make the dip: In a small, microwave-safe bowl, combine the peanut butter and chocolate chips. Heat on high in 15-second increments, stirring in between each, until the chocolate is melted. Remove from the microwave with an oven mitt.

2. Add the yogurt and fold the mixture into a fluffy mousse.

3. Choose a topping, if you'd like, and enjoy dipping your fruit into this scrumptious sweet treat.

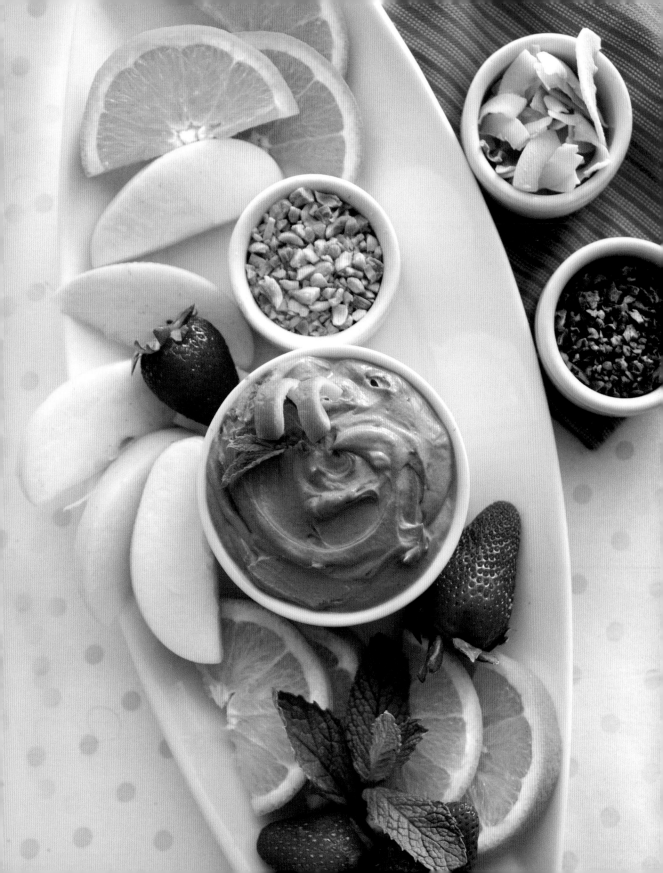

Easy Tortilla Chips

Makes 40 chips
Serving size: 5 chips
Per serving: calories 70; fat 2 g; fiber 2 g; protein 2 g; carbohydrates 11 g

---

Never again will you be out of tortilla chips. My skinny tortilla chips are easy to make and far better than the stuff you buy at the store. I buy whole wheat tortillas in bulk and store them in my freezer; they freeze beautifully and are flat, so they don't take up much space. Try them with Five-Minute Salsa (page 96) and Watermelon Margaritas (page 270) as shown here.

4 whole wheat tortillas
Olive oil spray
1 teaspoon kosher salt
½ teaspoon freshly ground black pepper

1. Preheat the oven to 350°F.

2. Lay the tortillas on a cutting board. Use a pizza wheel to slice each tortilla into ten wedges, like a pizza.

3. Spread out the chips on two rimmed baking sheets, spray them with olive oil, and sprinkle them with the salt and pepper. Bake for 10 to 15 minutes, or until the chips are crisp. Let them cool for 3 minutes on the baking sheets. Store in an airtight container or freezer bag at room temperature for 3 to 4 days.

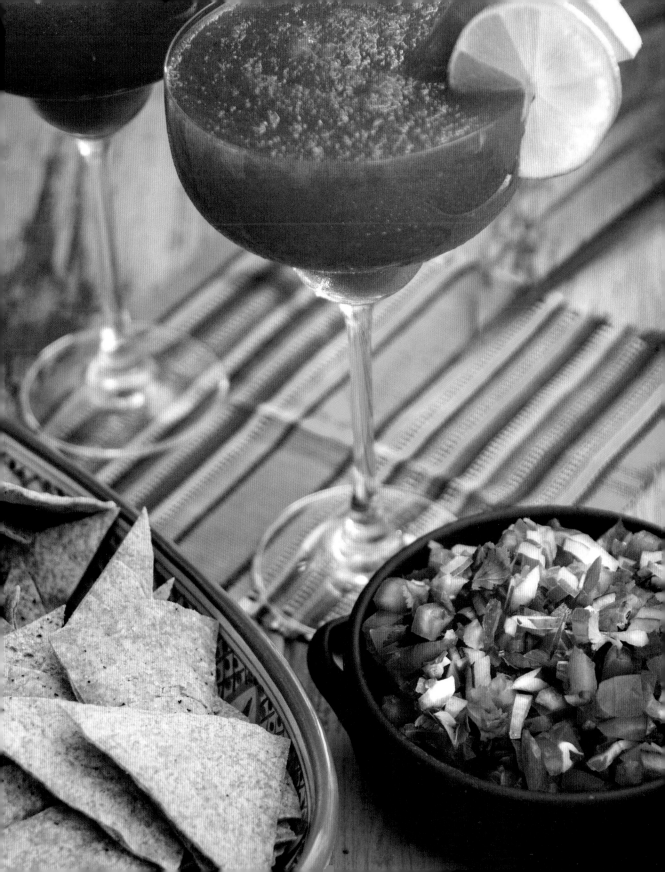

Rosemary Olive Oil Wheat Crackers

Makes 200 crackers
Serving size: 5 crackers
Per serving: calories 53; fat 2 g; fiber 1 g; protein 1 g; carbohydrates 8 g

I love these crackers—they taste just like Wheat Thins, but with only five ingredients. They're so much better for you, and cheaper, too! Chances are you have all these ingredients in your cabinet right now. Check out the variations below for optional flavors.

3 cups whole wheat flour, plus more
    for dusting
1 teaspoon kosher salt
⅓ cup extra-virgin olive oil
2 teaspoons finely chopped fresh rosemary
1 cup warm water

1. Preheat the oven to 350°F.

2. In the bowl of a stand mixer fitted with the dough hook attachment or in a bowl with a wooden spoon, combine all the ingredients and mix until you have a firm dough, about 3 minutes.

3. Divide the dough into four balls. On a floured surface, roll each ball into a large, very thin rectangle (be sure you get it as thin as you can), about 1½ feet long. Use a pizza wheel or knife to cut the dough into small 1-inch squares (or use cookie cutters for fun shapes) and place them on a rimmed baking sheet, sprinkling them with more salt, if desired.

4. Bake the crackers for 10 to 15 minutes, until crisp and golden brown. Let cool completely and store in an airtight bag or container for up to 1 week.

"Original" Wheat Crackers: Remove the rosemary and add ¼ teaspoon sugar.

Garlic Bread: Remove the rosemary and add 2 minced garlic cloves, 2 tablespoons grated Parmesan cheese, and 2 teaspoons dried parsley.

Sun-Dried Tomato Basil: Remove the rosemary and add 2 finely chopped sun-dried tomatoes and 2 tablespoons finely chopped fresh basil.

Cinnamon Sugar: Remove the rosemary and add 1 teaspoon ground cinnamon and 1 tablespoon sugar to the dough and sprinkle 1 teaspoon each cinnamon and sugar on top of the crackers before baking.

Rosemary Parmesan: Add 2 teaspoons grated Parmesan cheese.

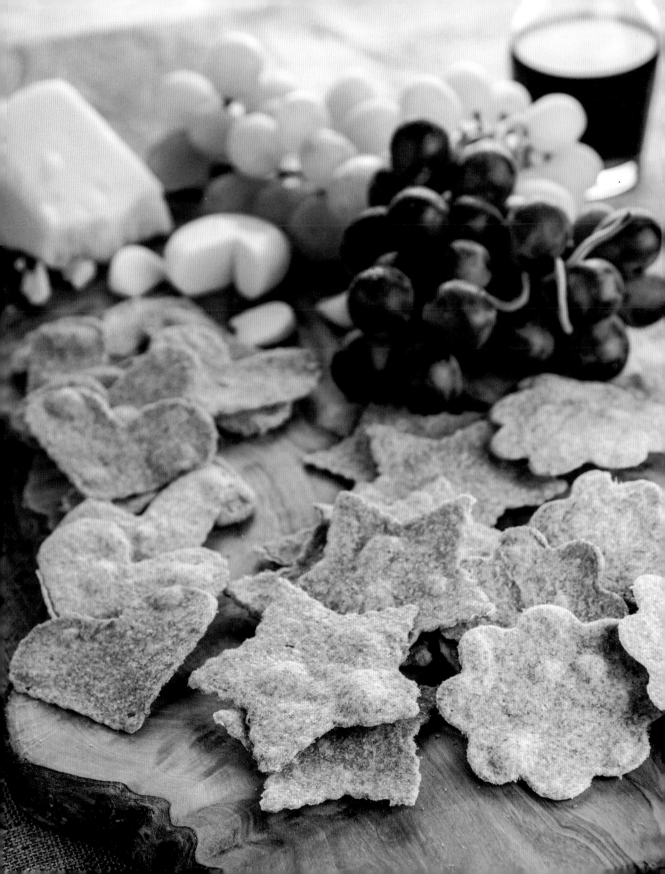

TWENTY-FIVE SNACKS
UNDER 100 CALORIES

Skip the store-bought 100-calorie snacks—they never satisfy and leave you full of preservatives and other chemicals that can negatively affect your weight loss. These twenty-five super-snacks will speed up your weight loss and leave you feeling much more satisfied. Plus, they're less expensive than the pricy prepackaged stuff.

1 cup blueberries (85 calories)

2 figs (75 calories)

1 hard-boiled egg (75 calories)

1 small baked sweet potato (55 calories)

1 medium apple (70 calories)

25 unsalted pistachios (85 calories)

13 whole almonds (90 calories)

⅓ cup shelled edamame (65 calories)

2 kiwis (95 calories)

2 cups watermelon chunks (90 calories)

1 cup raspberries (65 calories)

2 cups air-popped popcorn with 1 teaspoon butter (95 calories)

3 apricots (60 calories)

1 banana (55 calories)

½ cup (about 25) cherries (60 calories)

1½ cups cantaloupe chunks (80 calories)

½ mango (65 calories)

1 orange (60 calories)

1 peach (40 calories)

1 pear (50 calories)

½ papaya (60 calories)

1 cup fresh pineapple chunks (75 calories)

3 large carrots (90 calories)

2 cups strawberries (99 calories)

1 cucumber, sliced (50 calories)

· Chapter 7 ·

Pizza, Pizza

Yes, it's possible . . . you can lose weight eating pizza! You know you love me now! I cut hundreds of calories with just a few Smart Swaps, and I like to brag that I can make three pizzas for five dollars (depending on the toppings, of course). I like making these pizzas for *Monday Night Football*. I make the dough and sauce in the morning before leaving the house and let the dough rise all day. When I get home, I assemble the pizzas and cook, all in under twenty minutes. It's faster, cheaper, and healthier than delivery—just don't tell your family it's so easy or they'll ask for it every day.

My favorite Smart Swaps for this chapter:

Water! I use lots of water in the pizza dough so I don't have to use as much olive oil. It makes for a delicious, crispy crust and cuts hundreds of calories.

Turkey sausage and turkey pepperoni help cut hundreds of calories while boosting the flavor. Be sure to get nitrate-free!

Fresh herbs and garlic: I boost the flavor with lots of fresh herbs and garlic. No one ever notices that these are "skinny" recipes because they're so packed full of flavor.

Perfect Pizza Dough and Sauce

Makes 3 pizzas, 12 servings total
Serving size: 2 slices
Per serving: calories 161; fat 4 g; fiber 2 g; protein 4 g; carbohydrates 27 g

I love making homemade pizza, and during football season I make it weekly! My family has come to love this skinny version so much that it's always requested over ordering takeout. They love the taste, and I love the cost savings!

The dough and sauce recipes are enough for three pizzas, but the toppings in the following recipes are enough for one pizza. This allows for many different options. Should you want to make three of the same pizza, just triple those particular toppings.

Perfect Pizza Dough

1 (¼-ounce) package Fleischmann's
　　RapidRise yeast
1 cup warm water, plus more as needed
3¼ cups all-purpose flour, plus more
　　for dusting
1 teaspoon kosher salt
¼ cup olive oil
Medium-coarse cornmeal
　　(if using a pizza stone)

Perfect Pizza Sauce

1 (15-ounce) can tomato sauce
1 (6-ounce) can tomato paste
3 tablespoons chopped fresh basil
3 cloves garlic, finely chopped
⅛ teaspoon sugar
Kosher salt and freshly ground
　　black pepper

1. Make the dough: In a small bowl, dissolve the yeast in ¼ cup of the warm water. Set aside until it froths in the bowl.

2. In the bowl of a stand mixer fitted with the dough hook attachment or in a large bowl, combine the flour and salt. Make a well in the middle and pour in the yeast mixture, oil, and remaining ¾ cup warm water. Mix until a dough forms.

3. Knead for 5 minutes (you may need to add a little more warm water) until you have a firm dough that's slightly tacky but doesn't stick to your hands, if kneading with your hands (see my easy how-to directions on page 140).

4. Dust a large bowl with flour. Put the dough in the bowl and cover with plastic wrap and then a kitchen towel. Let the dough rise on your countertop for at least 2 hours, or until the dough has doubled in size.

5. Make the sauce: In a large glass jar or medium bowl, combine all the sauce ingredients. Mix well, cover, and let marinate on your kitchen counter while the dough rises, or leave it overnight in the fridge.

6. Preheat the oven to 500°F about 20 minutes before baking. (If you are using a pizza stone, place it in the oven at this time.)

7. Punch the dough down and knead it for 2 minutes. Divide it into three softball-size balls. Sprinkle a clean surface and rolling pin with flour and roll out the dough balls.

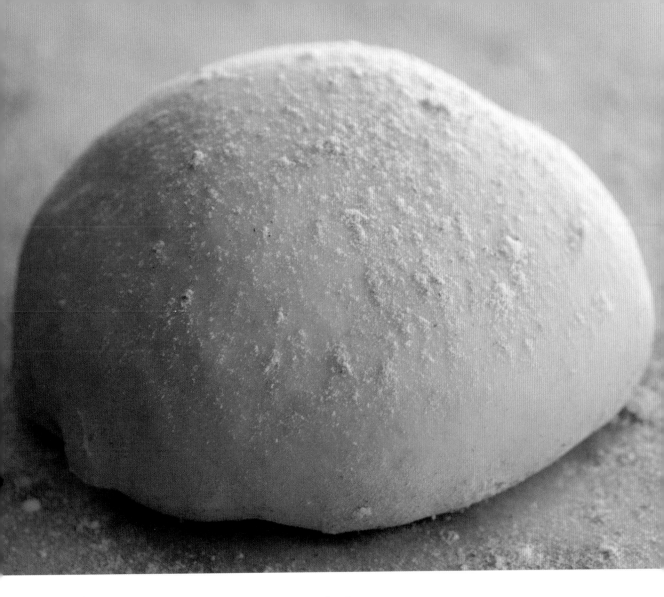

8. If you're using a pizza stone, sprinkle some cornmeal on a pizza peel. Transfer the rolled-out dough to a pizza pan, baking sheet, or prepared pizza peel.

9. Proceed with the following pizza recipe of your choice! To store extra dough for later, sprinkle flour over the dough ball and wrap it in waxed paper before placing it in a freezer bag. You can also place the extra sauce in a freezer bag. Store together in the fridge for 48 hours or in the freezer for up to 1 month.

NOTE: You can't hurt this dough. If it's too sticky, add some flour; if it's too dry, add more water. Just add slowly, no more than a tablespoon at a time.

Margherita Pizza

Makes 1 pizza, 8 slices
Serving size: 2 slices
Per serving: calories 218; fat 8 g; fiber 2 g; protein 5 g; carbohydrates 28 g

If you've never heard of Margherita pizza, you're probably a little confused—no, you don't blend this up and serve it with lime wedges. It's actually a very famous pizza named for a queen of Italy. In 1866, the tomato, basil, and mozzarella pizza was the most popular pizza in Naples. It was named for Queen Margherita of Savoy in 1889, mainly because she loved pizza but eating peasant food was taboo . . . so they named one for her. There's plenty of debate over its origins, but no one can deny how delicious it is!

I love how the basil adds brightness to this pizza. It's my personal favorite and a fun way to make a "cheese pizza" a little more chic and grown up. Check out my Guide to the Perfect Salad (page 18) or try a crisp Caesar salad with this. A Caesar and a queen on one plate—how fancy!

1 ball Perfect Pizza Dough (page 124)
½ cup Perfect Pizza Sauce (page 124)
⅓ cup grated mozzarella cheese
5 large or 8 small basil leaves
1 tomato, sliced

1. Preheat the oven to 500°F. Roll out the pizza dough as directed on page 124.

2. Spoon the sauce over the dough, sprinkle on the cheese, and top with the basil leaves and tomato slices. There is no right or wrong way to top this pizza. If you want to make a smiley face or stripes with the tomatoes and basil, do so. Have fun and enjoy topping your pizza, or have the kids do this part to get them excited about their food.

3. Place the pizza in the oven or slide it from the pizza peel or paddle onto the hot pizza stone. Bake for 10 minutes. Watch closely—if one side browns faster than the other, turn it halfway through. When the cheese has melted and the crust is golden, remove the pizza from the oven and let it sit for 3 minutes on the hot pan to continue cooking the bottom of the crust. If using a pizza stone, use the peel or paddle to remove the pizza to a cool countertop or cutting board.

4. Use a pizza wheel or scissors to cut the pizza into eight slices.

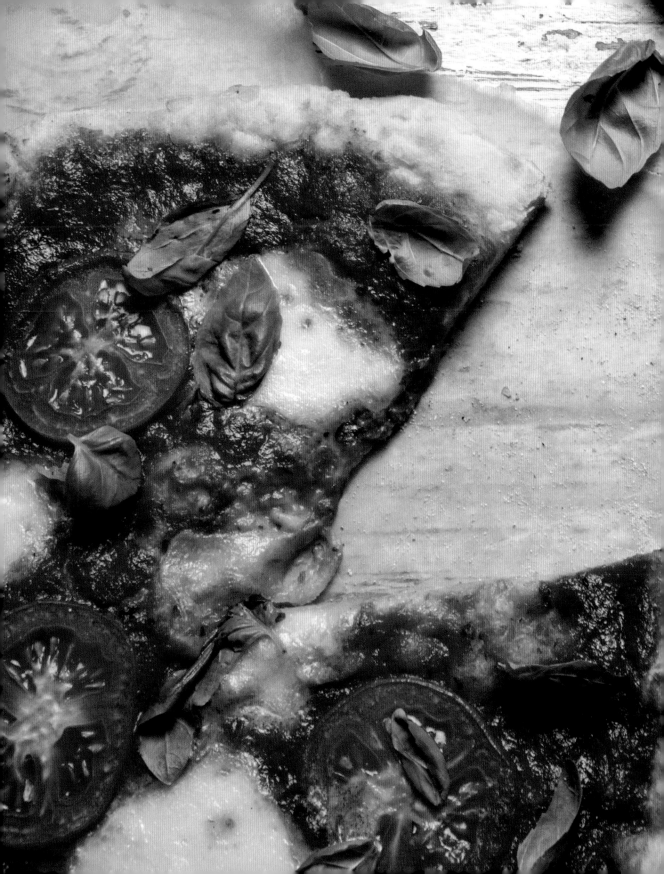

Sausage Mushroom Pizza

Makes 1 pizza, 8 slices
Serving size: 2 slices
Per serving: calories 235; fat 8 g; fiber 2 g; protein 7 g; carbohydrates 29 g

I love the combo of Italian sausage and sliced mushrooms on pizza. I cut the calories and fat by using turkey sausage. The mushrooms make this pizza seem even more meaty and delicious.

I live in wine country in California, and often I'm asked by local publications and wineries to create recipes that pair well with wine. I worked with a similar recipe and paired it with a reserve cabernet, although a merlot or bold red blend will pair beautifully and impress your guests or family. Here's a good wine rule of thumb: if you're not sure what to buy, get a red wine between fifteen and twenty dollars. That should guarantee you a solid wine; anything cheaper might be wasting your money.

1 ball Perfect Pizza Dough (page 124)
1 Italian turkey sausage, casing removed
½ cup Perfect Pizza Sauce (page 124)
⅓ cup grated mozzarella cheese
½ cup sliced white mushrooms
¼ red onion, thinly sliced

1. Preheat the oven to 500°F. Roll out the pizza dough as directed on page 124.

2. In a small skillet, cook the sausage over medium heat, crumbling it as it cooks, about 10 minutes. Drain on paper towels to remove some of the fat.

3. Spoon the sauce onto the dough. Sprinkle on the cheese, mushrooms, onion, and sausage.

4. Place the pizza in the oven or slide it from the pizza peel or paddle onto the hot pizza stone. Bake for 10 minutes, watching closely. If one side browns faster than the other, turn it halfway through. When the cheese has melted and the crust is golden, remove the pizza from the oven and let sit for 3 minutes on the hot pan to continue cooking the bottom of the crust. If using a pizza stone, use the peel or paddle to remove the pizza to a cool countertop or cutting board.

5. Use a pizza wheel or scissors to cut the pizza into eight slices.

It's easy to remove sausage casing: Cut the sausage casing down the length of the sausage with a sharp knife or scissors, then use your fingers or a wooden spoon to separate the meat from the outer casing. For easy cleanup, do this work in the pan before you heat it up. You can also slice the sausage crosswise into rounds, as shown here.

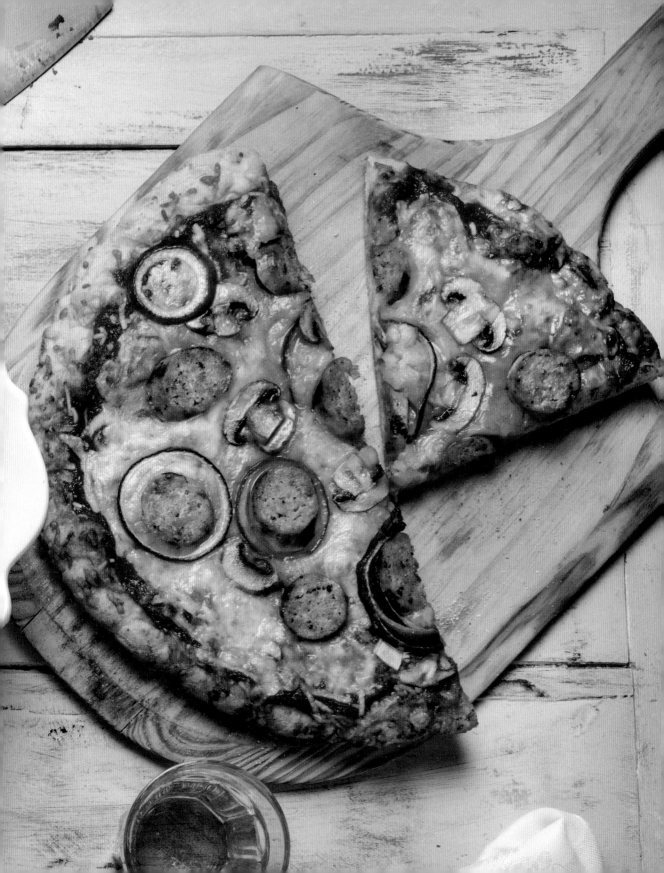

Supreme Pizza

Makes 1 pizza, 8 slices
Serving size: 2 slices
Per serving: calories 255; fat 9 g; fiber 2 g; protein 11 g; carbohydrates 34 g

Ask your family if they want a vegetarian pizza and they may say no. But if you offer to make a Supreme Pizza, they will cheer. Truth be told, it's the perfect combo of vegetables and meaty goodness. It's all in the delivery. That's how you get your family to eat more veggies.

If you don't use up all your toppings, add them to a freezer bag and toss it in the freezer. You'll have them chopped and ready for the next time you make this pizza.

1 ball Perfect Pizza Dough (page 124)
½ cup Perfect Pizza Sauce (page 124)
⅓ cup grated mozzarella cheese
1 small tomato, sliced
¼ cup sliced mushrooms
½ bell pepper, sliced into rings
¼ onion, thinly sliced
2 tablespoons sliced black olives
½ Italian turkey sausage, casing removed, cooked (see page 128)
2 tablespoons turkey pepperoni

1. Preheat the oven to 500°F. Roll out the pizza dough as directed on page 124.

2. Spoon the sauce onto the dough. Sprinkle on the cheese and top with the remaining ingredients.

3. Place the pizza in the oven or slide it from the pizza peel or paddle onto the hot pizza stone. Bake for 10 minutes, watching closely. If one side browns faster than the other, turn it halfway through. When the cheese has melted and the crust is golden, remove the pizza from the oven and let it sit for 3 minutes on the hot pan to continue cooking the bottom crust. If using a pizza stone, use the peel or paddle to remove the pizza to a cool countertop or cutting board.

4. Use a pizza wheel or scissors to cut the pizza into eight slices.

Vegetarian Pizza: Swap in ¼ cup sliced artichoke hearts for the sausage and pepperoni.

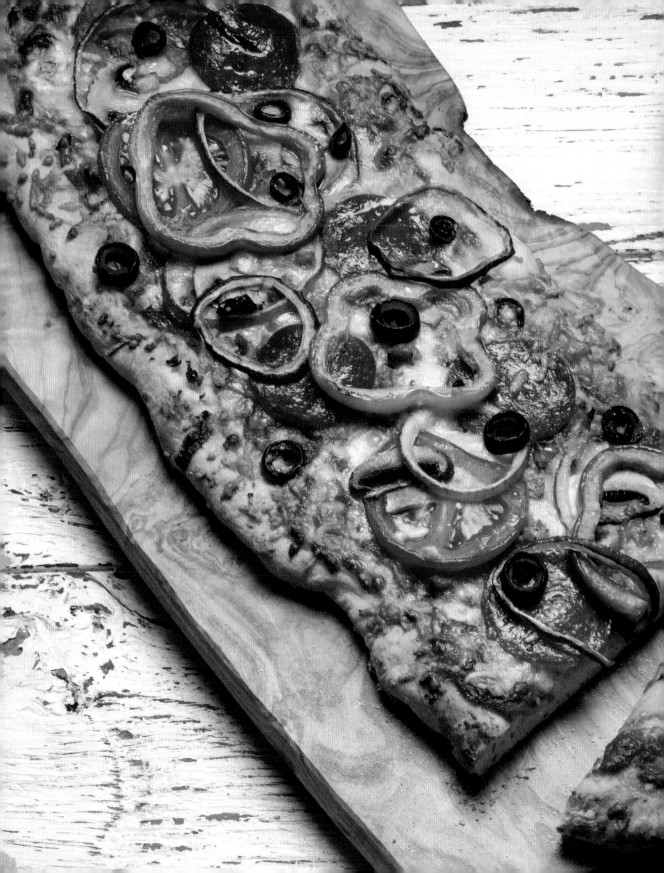

Hawaiian Pizza

Makes 1 pizza, 8 slices
Serving size: 2 slices
Per serving: calories 240; fat 8 g; fiber 2 g; protein 11 g; carbohydrates 31 g

This is my daughter's favorite pizza. She really loves pineapple! I get frozen, organic pineapple. The stuff in a can may last on shelves for years (yuck), but it's soaking in sugar. All I need to do is grab a handful or two from the bag of frozen pineapple and let it defrost in a bowl while the pizza dough rises.

If you use frozen pineapple, check out my Pineapple Mango Ginger Sorbet (page 252). It's the perfect sweet treat after this yummy pizza and a great way to feature leftover pineapple.

1 ball Perfect Pizza Dough (page 124)
½ cup Perfect Pizza Sauce (page 124)
⅓ cup shredded mozzarella cheese
⅓ cup chopped fresh or frozen pineapple
3 slices Canadian bacon,
   coarsely chopped
¼ red onion, thinly sliced

1. Preheat the oven to 500°F. Roll out the pizza dough as directed on page 124.

2. Spoon the sauce onto the dough and sprinkle on the cheese. Top with the remaining ingredients.

3. Place the pizza in the oven or slide it from the pizza peel or paddle onto the hot pizza stone. Bake for 10 minutes, watching closely. If one side browns faster than the other, turn it halfway through. When the cheese has melted and the crust is golden, remove the pizza from the oven and let it sit for 3 minutes on the hot pan to continue cooking the bottom crust. If using a pizza stone, use the peel or paddle to remove the pizza to a cool countertop or cutting board.

4. Use a pizza wheel or scissors to cut the pizza into eight slices.

Cowboy Pizza

Makes 1 pizza, 8 slices
Serving size: 2 slices
Per serving: calories 315; fat 14 g; fiber 2 g; protein 14.5 g; carbohydrates 32 g

Yee-haw, this is a delicious recipe! I use my Homemade Barbecue Sauce to spice up the chicken, but you can use any organic BBQ sauce you like. I also use leftover shredded chicken in this recipe; it helps keep the cost low and is a yummy way to use up leftovers.

1 ball Perfect Pizza Dough (page 124)
½ cup shredded cooked chicken
¼ cup plus 3 tablespoons Homemade
   Barbecue Sauce (page 170)
½ cup Perfect Pizza Sauce (page 124)
⅓ cup shredded mozzarella cheese
¼ red onion, thinly sliced
1 tomato, chopped
Sliced pickled jalapeños (optional)

1. Preheat the oven to 500°F. Roll out the pizza dough as directed on page 124.

2. In a small bowl, combine the chicken and ¼ cup of the barbecue sauce. Mix until all the chicken is coated.

3. Spoon the pizza sauce onto the dough and sprinkle on the cheese. Top with the chicken and onion.

4. Place the pizza in the oven or slide it from the pizza peel or paddle onto the hot pizza stone. Bake for 10 minutes, watching closely. If one side browns faster than the other, turn it halfway through. When the cheese has melted and the crust is golden, remove the pizza from the oven and let it sit for 3 minutes on the hot pan to continue cooking the bottom crust. If using a pizza stone, use the peel or paddle to remove the pizza to a cool countertop or cutting board.

5. Drizzle the remaining 3 tablespoons BBQ sauce on top and add the tomato and jalapeños, if using. Use a pizza wheel or scissors to cut the pizza into eight slices.

NOTE: If you don't have leftover chicken available, simply drizzle 1 teaspoon olive oil over a chicken breast, season with salt and pepper, and cook in a skillet over medium heat, turning once, until cooked through, about 10 minutes. Let rest for 5 to 10 minutes, then shred the chicken with two forks.

Pear, Rosemary, and Goat Cheese Pizza

Makes 1 pizza, 8 slices
Serving size: 2 slices
Per serving: calories 345; fat 13 g; fiber 3 g; protein 12 g; carbohydrates 49 g

One of my favorite wineries makes this pizza, and I've been told by the chef that the sprinkle of sea salt at the very end is the secret ingredient. I've made it without, and I can definitely taste the difference, so be sure you don't skip this step! And since this is from a winery, I feel I must tell you that this pizza pairs great with a crisp white wine like pinot gris, albariño, or chardonnay.

If you can't have cow's milk, you can swap all the cheeses for crumbled goat cheese.

Caramelized Onions
1 tablespoon olive oil
1 onion, sliced into thin rings
¼ teaspoon kosher salt

Pizza
1 ball Perfect Pizza Dough (page 124)
1 tablespoon extra-virgin olive oil
2 teaspoons finely chopped fresh rosemary
2 cloves garlic, thinly sliced
¼ cup mozzarella cheese
1 pear, cored and thinly sliced
2 tablespoons crumbled goat cheese
2 tablespoons grated Parmesan cheese
1 teaspoon sea salt

1. Make the caramelized onions: In a large sauté pan, heat the olive oil over medium-low heat. Add the onion and salt and cook, stirring often, until the onion is soft and caramelized, about 1 hour.

2. Make the pizza: Preheat the oven to 500°F. Roll out the pizza dough as directed on page 124.

3. Drizzle the olive oil over the crust. Sprinkle the dough with the rosemary and garlic. Top with the mozzarella, pear, goat cheese, and Parmesan.

4. Place the pizza in the oven or slide it from the pizza peel or paddle onto the hot pizza stone. Bake for 10 minutes, watching closely. If one side browns faster than the other, turn it halfway through. When the cheese has melted and the crust is golden, remove the pizza from the oven and let it sit for 3 minutes on the hot pan to continue cooking the bottom crust. If using a pizza stone, use the peel or paddle to remove the pizza to a cool countertop or cutting board.

5. Top with the caramelized onions and sprinkle on the sea salt. Use a pizza wheel or scissors to cut the pizza into eight slices.

NOTE: If you want to make your caramelized onions even more flavorful, add 2 coarsely chopped garlic cloves and 1 sprig of fresh thyme to the onions and cook as directed, removing and discarding the thyme sprig when you are through cooking. Then give them a single dash of Worcestershire sauce.

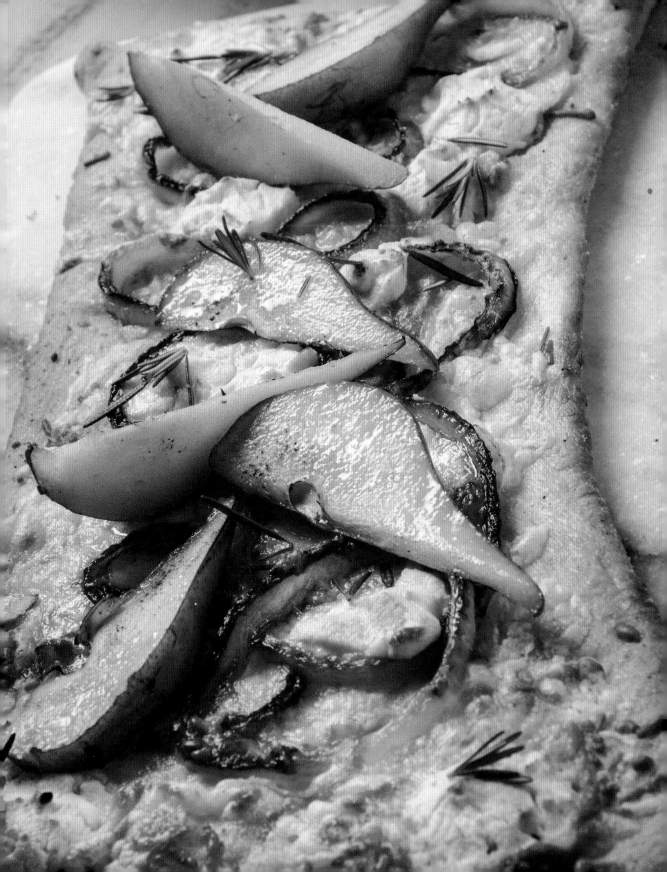

California Club Pizza

Makes 1 pizza, 8 slices
Serving size: 2 slices
Per serving: calories 262; fat 11 g; fiber 1 g; protein 10 g; carbohydrates 32 g

Any excuse to eat avocados and I'm in. This pizza is full of veggies and it's a great way to mix it up on pizza night. Make this alongside the Sausage Mushroom Pizza (page 128) and you'll feel like you're eating at a fancy pizza parlor. If you're in a rush, you can make this on a whole wheat pita—see the variations below for cooking directions.

Choose homemade Ranch Salad Dressing over store-bought. The expensive store-bought stuff is full of chemicals that impede weight loss. But my skinny ranch is all natural, low calorie, low cost, and made with some metabolism-boosting ingredients to actually help you lose weight.

1 ball Perfect Pizza Dough (page 124)
1 slice bacon
1 tablespoon olive oil
¼ cup grated mozzarella cheese
2 cloves garlic, minced
¼ red onion, thinly sliced
1 avocado, pitted, peeled, and cut into
    ½-inch chunks
1 tomato, chopped
¼ cup Ranch Salad Dressing (page 105)
2 tablespoons grated Parmesan cheese

1. Preheat the oven to 500°F. Roll out the pizza dough as directed on page 124.

2. In a skillet, cook the bacon over medium heat until it's as crispy as you like it. Move to a paper towel–lined plate to cool, then crumble and set aside.

3. Drizzle the olive oil over the crust. Sprinkle the mozzarella over the dough and top with the garlic and red onion.

4. Place the pizza in the oven or slide it from the pizza peel or paddle onto the hot pizza stone. Bake for 10 minutes, watching closely. If one side browns faster than the other, turn it halfway through. When the cheese has melted and the crust is golden, remove the pizza from the oven and let it sit for 3 minutes on the hot pan to continue cooking the bottom crust. If using a pizza stone, use the peel or paddle to transfer the pizza to a cool countertop or cutting board.

5. Top with the bacon, avocado, and tomato. Drizzle with the ranch dressing and sprinkle with the Parmesan cheese. Use a pizza wheel or scissors to cut the pizza into eight slices.

For an individual-size pizza, use a whole wheat pita, top as directed, and bake for 5 to 8 minutes.

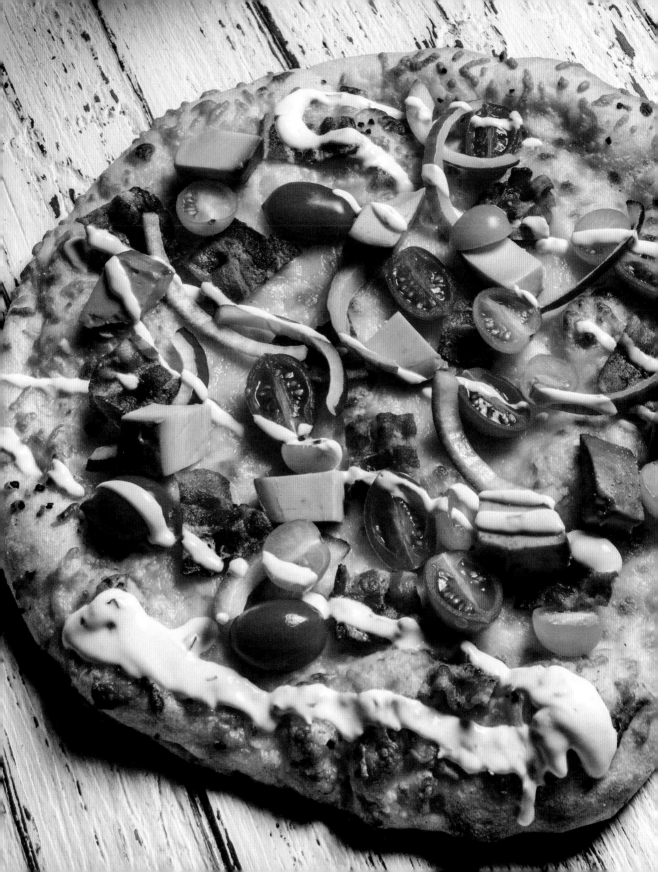

Pizza Rolls

Makes 4 rolls (32 slices)
Serving size: 2 slices
Per serving: calories 202; fat 7 g; fiber 2 g; protein 9 g; carbohydrates 24 g

I used to frequent a lovely Italian restaurant in Orange County, California, known for its namesake dish, Peppino Bread. This incredible rolled pizza/calzone with pizza sauce for dipping is out of sight! I couldn't think of a life without this dish, so I created a skinny version—one I could make whenever I liked without guilt.

These are great for potlucks. They travel well and are good hot or at room temperature. They're the perfect finger food for football-watching parties, too. Sometimes I even make them for dinner with a crisp green salad just so I can enjoy the leftovers the next day at lunch.

If you have a vegetarian in your home, you can make one or more of these pizza rolls without meat; see below for vegetarian options.

1 recipe Perfect Pizza Dough (page 124), with 1 teaspoon garlic powder added to the flour
1 (8-ounce) ball mozzarella cheese, shredded
1 cup organic nitrate-free turkey pepperoni
10 fresh basil leaves
1 recipe Perfect Pizza Sauce (page 124)

1. Preheat the oven to 450°F.

2. When the dough has risen, punch it down and knead again for 1 minute. Divide the dough into four balls. On a clean, floured surface, roll out each dough ball into a 9 x 13-inch rectangle, working one at a time.

3. Over each rectangle of dough, spread ¼ cup of the shredded mozzarella cheese, ¼ cup of the pepperoni, and some basil leaves. Leave an inch of bare dough along the sides.

4. Working on the widest side, fold the bottom half up and the top down over the first fold so you are left with a long roll. Move to a rimmed baking sheet, flipping so that the seam is on the bottom. Proceed to make the other three rolls.

5. Bake the rolls for 8 minutes, flip them over, and bake for 5 to 8 minutes more, or until golden brown on the top and edges.

6. While the rolls are baking, in a small saucepan, heat the sauce over medium-high heat until bubbling hot.

7. Use a pizza wheel to cut the pizza rolls crosswise, like a sushi roll, into eight pieces per roll. Serve with a bowl of hot pizza sauce for dipping.

Vegetarian Pizza Rolls: Use ½ cup of your favorite veggies in place of the pepperoni. Choose the veggies you prefer on your pizza—mushrooms, red onion, and olives are my favorites in these pizza rolls.

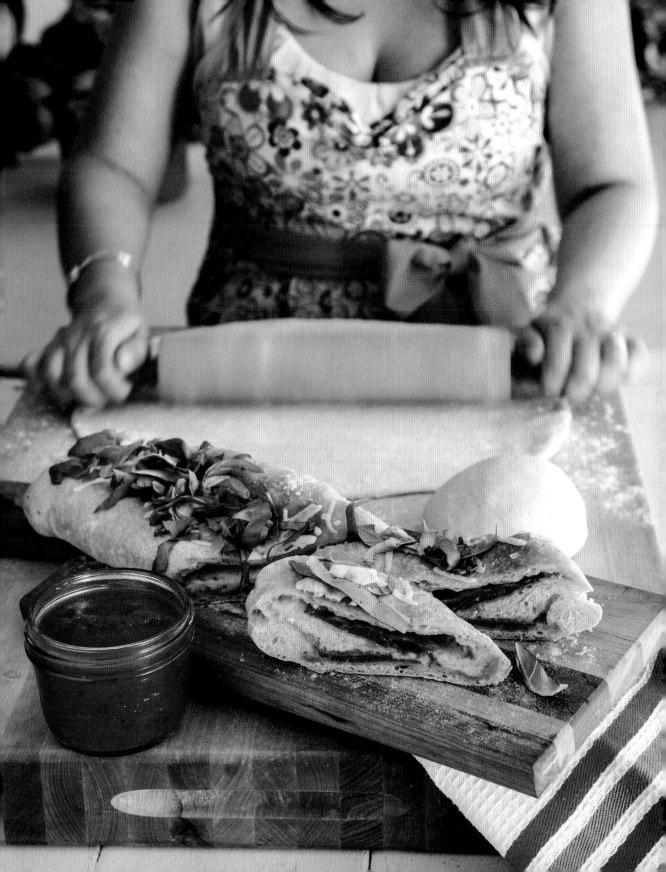

Pizza Bites

Makes 54 pizza bites
Serving size: 1 pizza bite
Per serving: calories 64; fat 2.5 g; fiber 1 g; protein 3 g;
carbohydrates 7 g (nutrition is based on all the toppings added)

Kids love those frozen pizza bites, but they're filled with preservatives and other chemicals, plus they're empty calories. Try this healthy and delicious version that kids love to eat and love to help make, too! They're great for kids' sleepovers, adult cocktail parties, and Sunday afternoon football with the family. Freeze leftovers in a large freezer bag, and you have microwavable pizza bites you can feel good about making for your kids.

Olive oil spray
1 (¼-ounce) package Fleischmann's RapidRise yeast
1 cup warm water
1½ cups all-purpose flour, plus more for dusting
1½ cups whole wheat flour
1 teaspoon kosher salt
¼ cup olive oil
1 recipe Perfect Pizza Sauce (page 124)
2 cups grated mozzarella cheese
1 Italian chicken or turkey sausage, casing removed, cooked and crumbled (see page 128) (optional)
1 bell pepper, chopped (optional)
8 button mushrooms, chopped (optional)
½ onion, chopped (optional)
1 large sprig fresh basil, torn into small pieces (optional)

1. In a small bowl, dissolve the yeast in ¼ cup of the warm water.

2. In the bowl of a stand mixer fitted with the dough hook attachment or in a large bowl with a spatula, combine both flours and the salt. Add the yeast mixture, oil, and remaining ¾ cup warm water. Turn the mixer on and knead for 4 minutes, or use a spatula to combine. (If you're mixing by hand, turn the dough out onto a clean, floured surface and knead for 5 to 8 minutes, until the dough is smooth and warm. You may need to add more warm water as you go. Kneading is easy—make a loose fist and push the dough out away from you. Fold over and repeat.)

3. Dust a large bowl with flour. Transfer the dough to the floured bowl and cover it with plastic wrap and a kitchen towel. Let the dough rise for 2 to 4 hours on your countertop, until it's more than doubled in size.

4. While the dough rises, make the Perfect Pizza Sauce.

5. Preheat the oven to 450°F. Lightly coat two or three mini-muffin pans with olive oil spray.

6. Punch down the dough to deflate it, then knead the dough for another minute and divide it into three softball-size balls. Cover a clean surface and rolling pin with flour and roll out the dough balls into 6 x 12-inch rectangles. With a pizza wheel, cut each one twice across the length of the rectangle and five times down the width of the rectangle, creating eighteen squares.

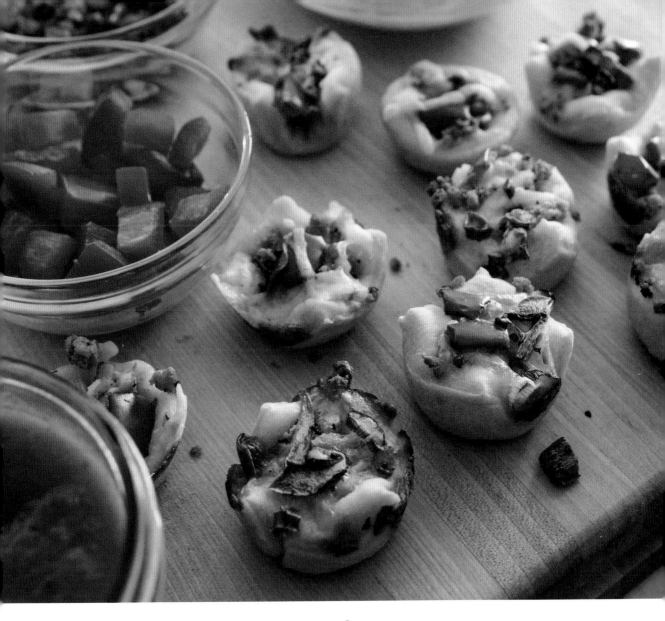

7. Place each square in a muffin cup. Top each with 1½ teaspoons of the sauce, about 1 teaspoon of the cheese, and ½ teaspoon of your desired toppings. (If you'd like, you can double up the toppings by adding ½ teaspoon under the cheese and ½ teaspoon on top.)

8. Bake for 8 to 12 minutes, or until the cheese has melted and browned and the bottoms of the pizza bites are golden brown. Let them cool in the tins before serving—this will help the bottoms crisp up.

NOTE: Prepare the sauce 2 hours ahead of assembling the pizza bites for the best flavor.

French Bread Pizza

Makes 16 slices
Serving size: 2 slices
Per serving: calories 278; fat 8g; fiber 2g; protein 17g; carbohydrates 34g

Here's a pizza recipe you can shop for in a flash and pull together in just twenty minutes on a weeknight. Look for a wide French bread loaf in the bakery section of your grocery store, or stop by a local bakery for fresh-baked goodness.

I cut the loaf horizontally in thirds and save the middle section for homemade croutons, eliminating a third of the bread and thus a third of the carbohydrates. I like to serve this with a crisp spring mix salad (see my Guide to the Perfect Salad on page 18)—you'll fill up and get your veggies, too.

1 (15-ounce) can tomato sauce
1 (6-ounce) can tomato paste
Leaves from 1 bunch fresh basil
    (about 25 leaves)
2 cloves garlic, chopped
1 tablespoon Italian seasoning
Pinch of sugar
Kosher salt and freshly ground
    black pepper
1 large French bread loaf
1 cup shredded mozzarella cheese
¼ cup organic nitrate-free turkey pepperoni

1. Preheat the oven to 370°F.

2. In a medium saucepan, whisk together the tomato sauce, tomato paste, basil, garlic, Italian seasoning, sugar, and salt and pepper to taste. Cover the pan and bring the mixture to a boil over medium heat, then take the pan off the heat.

3. Slice the bread horizontally in thirds, cutting off the top third and the bottom third. Reserve the middle third of the bread for croutons (page 72).

4. Place the top and bottom of the bread cut side up on a rimmed baking sheet. Spread half the hot pizza sauce evenly over each piece of bread. Sprinkle with the cheese and top with the pepperoni.

5. Bake for 15 to 20 minutes, until the cheese has melted and the bread is golden and crispy along the edges.

6. Let the pizza cool for 3 minutes before slicing. Cut each pizza into eight slices and serve with a fresh salad.

NOTE: Freeze half of this recipe before you bake it for an even quicker meal later. Wrap an uncooked French Bread Pizza in parchment paper and place in a freezer bag and freeze for up to 4 months. Defrost in your fridge and follow the baking directions, or bake from frozen by adding 10 to 15 minutes to the baking time.

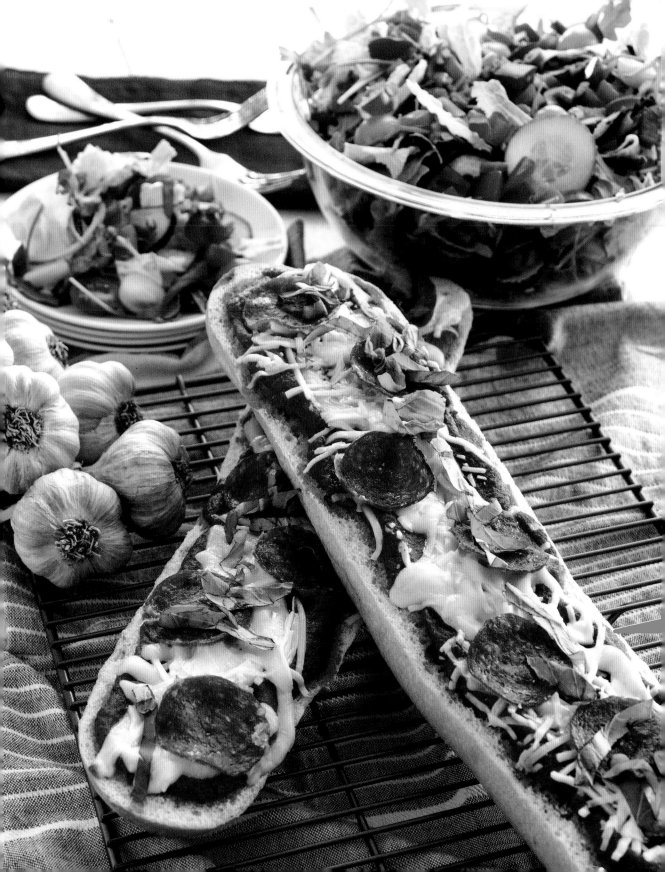

Chapter 8

Pasta Lovers

Alfredo and lasagna and meatballs, oh my! As an Italian American, I adore pasta and could never give it up, so I had to find healthier ways to eat it. First things first: Whole wheat pasta will keep you fuller longer, and once you put sauce on it, you can't tell the difference. Second, I snuck lots of veggies into these recipes. For instance, the lasagna is half veggies, but only the cook will know that.

There are all kinds of diets out there that recommend you remove all pasta from all meals, but humans have been eating carbohydrates and pasta for many years, and only in the last ten to fifteen years have people started removing these foods from their diets. In those same ten to fifteen years, the average weight in humans has risen to the heaviest ever. Demonizing foods and removing important food groups is not the way to go; eating all natural is. Think about it this way—if it's something your ancestors would have recognized as food, it's probably safe. If not, then steer clear. Try to find organic whole wheat pasta, since it is the closest thing to how our ancestors made and ate pasta.

My favorite Smart Swaps for this chapter:

Hidden veggies: I double up on onions, bell peppers, and any other veggies I can in these recipes. The veggies help you fill up while trimming down and stretch out recipes to feed more people (or produce more handy leftovers).

Turkey sausage tastes exactly the same as its full-fat cousins in recipes like these. Unless you are a sausage connoisseur, you'll never know the difference, but you will be shaving off hundreds of calories and loads of fat.

Chopped mushrooms mimic the heartiness of meat when cooked, soaking up the flavors around them.

Skinny Chicken Alfredo

Makes 10 servings
Serving size: about 1 cup
Per serving: calories 242; fat 4 g; fiber 2 g; protein 12 g; carbohydrates 39 g

Once you see how easy this Alfredo sauce is, you'll never buy premade again. I cut the fat and calories by reducing the amount of butter and flour and, of course, by swapping heavy cream with 1% milk. In truth, you can use whatever milk you have on hand, although with almond, coconut, or skim milk, it will take much more milk and time to thicken it up.

Use freshly grated block Parmesan cheese to make this dish. The canned or pregrated stuff won't give you the maximum sharp flavor you crave when you want Alfredo sauce. The sharper the cheese, the less you have to use, so invest in the good stuff. A little goes a long way, and it will last for ages in your fridge.

If you have a pepper grinder, opt for freshly ground pepper—it makes this dish so delicious.

1 (16-ounce) package whole wheat
    fettuccine pasta
1 boneless, skinless chicken breast
2 teaspoons olive oil
Kosher salt and freshly ground
    black pepper
2 tablespoons unsalted butter
2 tablespoons all-purpose flour
3 cups 1% milk
1 clove garlic
2 cups broccoli florets
5 tablespoons freshly grated Parmesan
    cheese

1. Bring a large saucepan of water to a boil. Add the pasta and cook until al dente according to the package directions. Drain and set aside.

2. Heat a skillet over medium-high heat. Drizzle the chicken with the olive oil, sprinkle with salt and pepper, add to the pan, and cook for 5 minutes on each side, until the center is no longer pink. Transfer to a plate to rest. Chop the chicken into cubes and set aside.

3. In a large saucepan, melt the butter over medium-low heat. Whisk in the flour. Cook, whisking, until the mixture browns and becomes a thick paste, about 5 minutes (this is the roux). Add the milk and garlic and cook, stirring, until the sauce just coats the back of your spoon, about 20 minutes. Transfer half the cream sauce to a bowl and set aside.

4. Remove the garlic clove from the sauce and discard it. Add the broccoli and cook for 5 minutes. Add the pasta, chicken, and pepper to the sauce and mix well so every piece of pasta is coated.

5. Remove the pasta from the heat and serve. Drizzle the extra sauce and ½ tablespoon Parmesan over each serving.

NOTE: I keep the quantity of chicken low to save money and calories, plus there's loads of protein in the sauce. But if you want to add more chicken, go for it. Each chicken breast you add to this dish will add 12 calories and 2 grams of protein per serving.

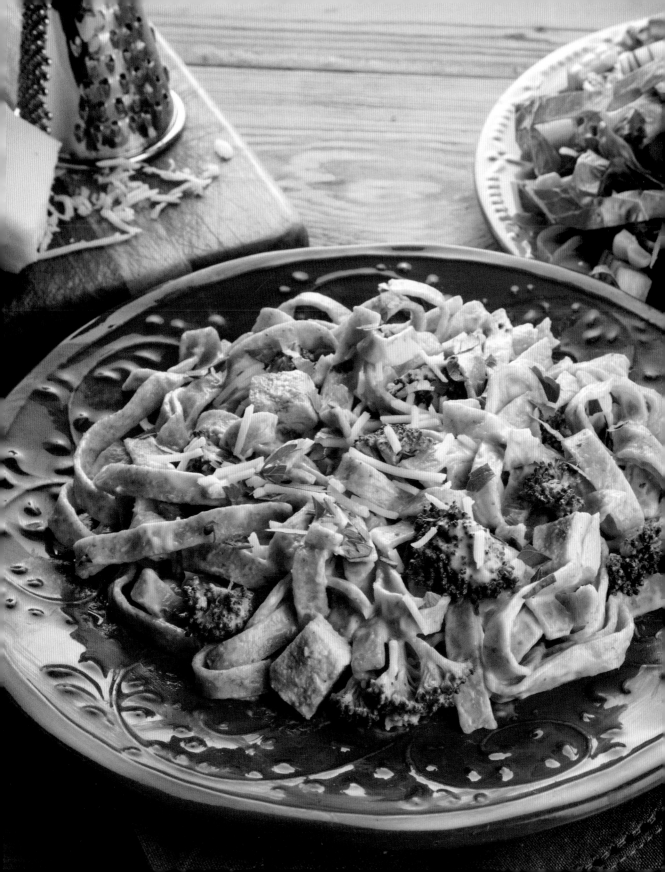

Meat Lovers' Baked Ziti

Makes 8 servings
Serving size: about 1 cup
Per serving: calories 352; fat 8 g; fiber 7 g; protein 21 g; carbohydrates 60 g

---

Baked ziti was a staple in my mom's house growing up, and it's become a staple in my house, too. This hearty baked pasta dish is perfect served with a crisp green salad on cold, rainy days. Make a big tray on Sunday nights for dinner and pack up the leftovers into individual "frozen meals" for fast weekday lunches and dinners.

I say this with much hesitation, but you can make this with an all-natural jarred tomato sauce. While I believe this dish is so delicious partly because of the fantastic marinara sauce I make it with, I can appreciate that you may not always have the time to make a batch of homemade sauce (although I strongly recommend you do and freeze it for this occasion). If you choose to use a jarred sauce, add some fresh basil or a couple dashes of Italian seasoning to kick it up a notch.

You may want to go for low-fat cheese here, but be aware that the fat in the cheese is needed for it to melt. If you use low-fat cheese it might taste good, but you'll end up with crispy cheese twigs rather than a melted cheese topping. Go for low-moisture mozzarella here; it's worth a few extra calories, and just a little goes a long way to creamy cheesy goodness.

1 (16-ounce) package whole wheat ziti
    or penne pasta
2 Italian chicken or turkey sausages
3 cups Slow-Cooker Marinara (page 159)
1 cup shredded mozzarella cheese
Handful of fresh parsley, chopped

1. Preheat the oven to 350°F.

2. Bring a large saucepan of water to a boil. Add the pasta and cook until al dente according to the package directions (it will continue to cook in the oven). Drain the pasta, return it to the pan, and set it aside.

3. In a large skillet, cook the sausages over medium-high heat. When the outsides start to brown, add the marinara sauce, cover, and bring to a boil. Reduce the heat to low and simmer for 15 minutes, or until the sausages are cooked through.

4. Remove the sausages from the sauce and transfer them to a plate. Use a fork and knife to chop them into small chunks, but be careful—they will be hot.

5. Add two-thirds of the marinara sauce to the pasta and mix to coat all the pasta. Transfer the pasta to a 9 x 13-inch casserole dish. Top it with the crumbled sausage, the remaining marinara sauce, and the shredded cheese.

6. Bake for 10 to 15 minutes, or until the cheese has melted and the edges start to crisp and brown.

7. Top the casserole with the parsley and let it rest for 5 minutes. (Letting it rest will help it hold together when you slice it.) Slice the casserole in half lengthwise, then slice across three times to make eight servings.

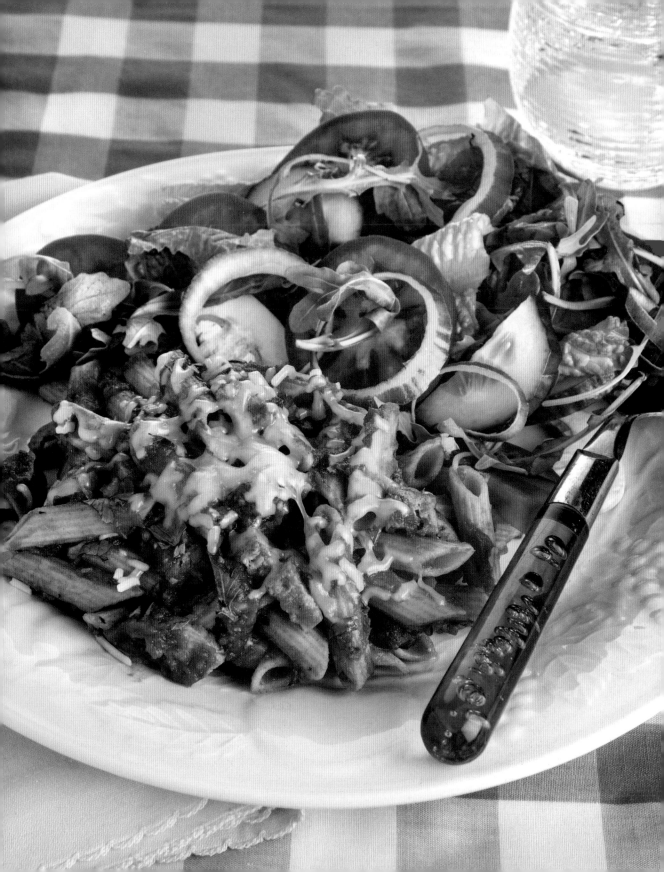

Spaghetti Bolognese

Makes 8 servings
Serving size: 1 cup spinach, ½ cup pasta, and ½ cup sauce
Per serving: calories 370; fat 8 g; fiber 10 g; protein 23 g; carbohydrates 59 g

I really love a good meat sauce, and this one freezes beautifully for leftovers. It also goes great with the Meat Lovers' Baked Ziti (page 148).

You might say this is a curious way to make a meat sauce, but I've found if you add the meat in the beginning, it becomes too dense and the meat falls apart. You want small chunks of meat in the end, so basically you make a delicious marinara sauce, and then at the last minute turn it into a Bolognese, making this a great slow cooker option and even a weeknight meal.

I know it may seem strange to add spinach, but it's so delicious and gives a boost of protein and fiber. I've become so fond of this metabolism-increasing ingredient that I can't imagine a red sauce without it. Even my husband, the quintessential meat-and-potatoes man, loves spinach in this and is always disappointed if I skip it. Just try it—I promise you'll love it! Covering spinach in Bolognese sauce is my all-time favorite way to eat it.

1 large yellow onion, finely chopped
4 cloves garlic, chopped
2 tablespoons Italian seasoning
1 tablespoon olive oil
¼ teaspoon kosher salt, plus more to taste
1 (28-ounce) can crushed tomatoes
1 (15-ounce) can tomato sauce
1 (6-ounce) can tomato paste
⅛ teaspoon sugar
Freshly ground black pepper
1 pound lean ground turkey
1 (16-ounce) package whole wheat spaghetti
8 cups baby spinach
Freshly grated Parmesan cheese, for serving

1. In a small bowl, combine 2 tablespoons of the onion and one-quarter of the chopped garlic. Add 1 tablespoon of the Italian seasoning to the bowl, cover, and set aside.

2. In a large saucepan, heat the olive oil over medium heat. Add the remaining onion and garlic, sprinkle with the salt, and cook, stirring to avoid burning, until the onion is soft and transparent, about 10 minutes. Mix in the remaining 1 tablespoon Italian seasoning and cook for 2 minutes, then add the crushed tomatoes, tomato sauce, tomato paste, sugar (to cut the acid in the tomatoes), and a sprinkling of salt and pepper to taste. Cook for 4 hours, stirring often to avoid burning. (Alternatively, cook the sauce in a slow cooker according to the directions on page 159.)

3. Heat a large skillet over medium-high heat. Brown the turkey with the onion-garlic mixture, about 10 minutes. Drain off any fat and add 1 cup of the cooked tomato sauce to the skillet. Cover and simmer for 20 minutes.

4. Meanwhile, bring a large saucepan of water to a boil. Add the spaghetti and cook until al dente according to the package directions. Drain the spaghetti (do not rinse it) and return it to the pan. Add 1 cup of the cooked tomato sauce and toss well to coat the pasta thoroughly.

5. Add the turkey mixture to the pot of tomato sauce and mix well.

6. To serve, spread 1 cup baby spinach on each plate. Top each with ½ cup of the pasta and ½ cup of the meat sauce. Sprinkle on a little Parmesan and enjoy.

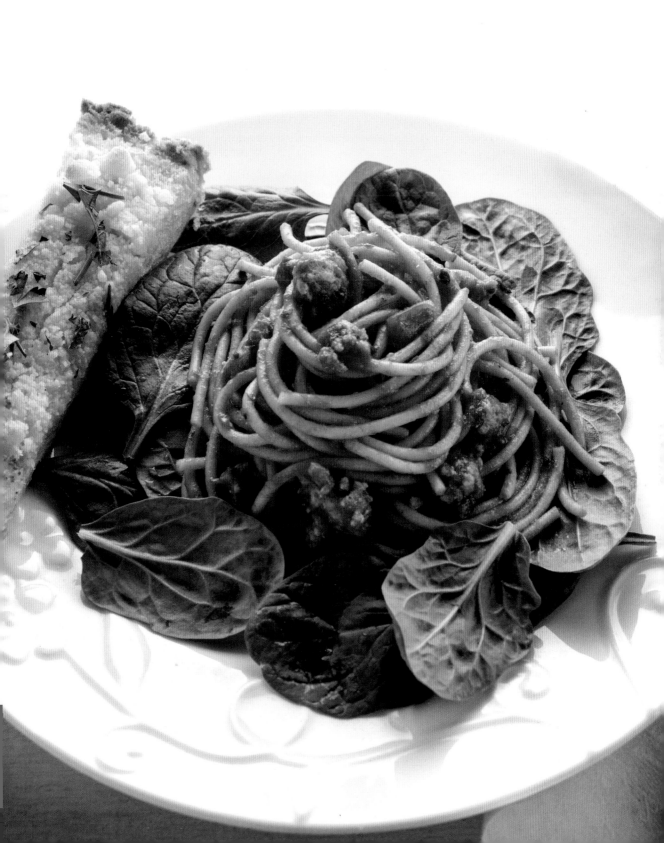

Greek Pasta Salad

Makes 15 servings
Serving size: about ½ cup
Per serving: calories 185; fat 7 g; fiber 2.5 g; protein 6 g; carbohydrates 27 g

I'm all for old-fashioned and even a bit kitschy, but I think traditional pasta salad needs a serious makeover! This new, hip pasta salad is packed full of bold, delicious flavors. It's fast and easy and can be served hot or cold, although I find that it's best at room temperature. Try this at your next potluck or barbecue and save your leftovers for lunches and side dishes. I serve leftovers over a plate of mixed greens, topped with a dollop of Tzatziki Dip (page 106). Yum yum!

I originally made this with gluten-free pasta to accommodate a guest, and it was so delicious I left the recipe alone. You can absolutely use any pasta you choose. Just try to use whole wheat at the very least—you can't tell the difference, so you might as well get an extra boost of nutrition.

I love to serve this alongside the Lemony Drumsticks (page 172) for the perfect picnic meal, and with the Strawberry Shortcake Cupcakes (page 246) for dessert, that's a 458-calorie meal including dessert!

Dressing
Zest of 1 lemon
Juice of 2 lemons
2 cloves garlic, minced
2 tablespoons spicy brown or Dijon mustard
3 tablespoons white balsamic vinegar
¼ cup extra-virgin olive oil
1 tablespoon juice from a jar of
    Kalamata olives
Kosher salt and freshly ground
    black pepper

Pasta
1 (12-ounce) box gluten-free penne or fusilli
    pasta, or any pasta you choose
1 pint cherry tomatoes, halved
15 Kalamata olives, sliced into thin rings
1 cucumber, cut into small chunks
½ red onion, roughly chopped
Handful of fresh parsley, chopped
1 cup crumbled low-fat feta cheese

1. Make the dressing: Make the dressing as early as you can, up to 24 hours beforehand. In a jar or medium bowl, combine all the dressing ingredients. Whisk well and refrigerate until you need it.

2. Bring a large saucepan of water to a boil. Add the pasta and cook until al dente according to the package directions. Drain.

3. While the pasta cooks, combine the tomatoes, olives, cucumber, and onion in a large bowl. Add the pasta, two-thirds of the parsley, and the dressing to the bowl and toss together.

4. Transfer to a serving dish, top with the crumbled feta and the remaining parsley, and serve.

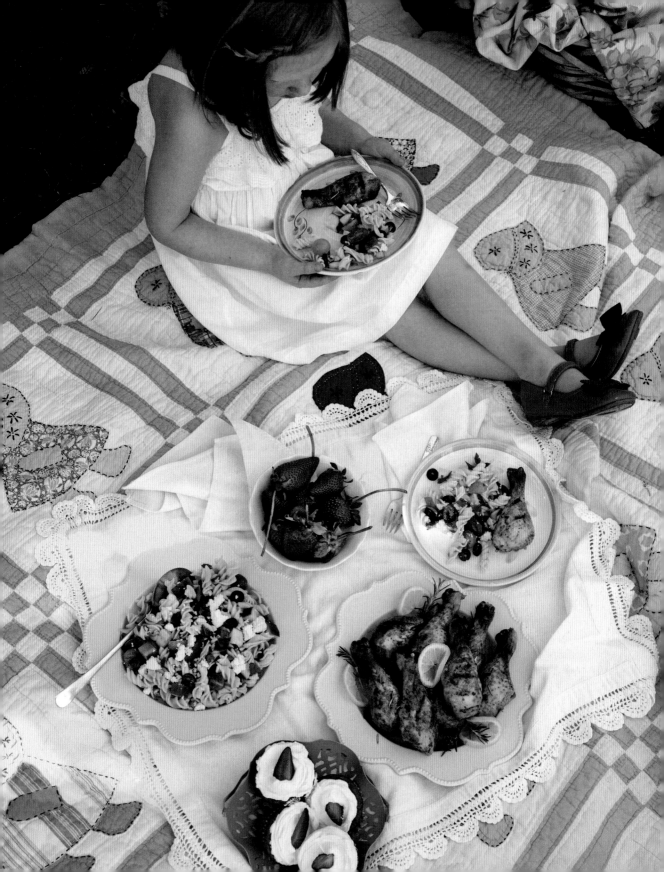

Vegetarian Stuffed Shells

Makes 35 stuffed shells
Serving size: 1 shell
Per serving: calories 73; fat 1.5 g; fiber 1 g; protein 3 g; carbohydrates 14 g

These stuffed shells are great for dinner parties, cocktail parties, and even weeknight family dinners! This recipe makes 35 shells, but you can easily cut the ingredients in half for a smaller portion.

Both Slow-Cooker Marinara and Bolognese (page 150) go great with these shells. It's a great way to use up leftovers and save money.

1 (12-ounce) box jumbo shells
2 teaspoons olive oil
1 onion, finely chopped
2 red bell peppers, finely chopped
2 cups mushrooms, chopped
2 cloves garlic, minced
Kosher salt and freshly ground
    black pepper
2 tablespoons Italian seasoning
½ cup low-fat ricotta cheese
3 cups Slow-Cooker Marinara (page 159)
½ cup shredded mozzarella cheese

1. In a large saucepan, bring 5 to 6 cups water to a boil. Add the shells and boil for 9 minutes, stirring occasionally. Drain and set the shells aside to cool. (I often do this the night or morning before I'm serving the shells and keep them in the fridge for easy handling.)

2. In a large sauté pan, heat the olive oil over medium heat. Add the onion, bell pepper, mushrooms, garlic, and a pinch of salt and pepper and stir to combine. Cook, stirring often to avoid burning, until the onion softens, about 10 minutes. Reduce the heat to medium-low and stir in the Italian seasoning. Cook to toast the herbs a bit, 1 to 2 minutes, or until fragrant. Set the pan aside to cool for 10 minutes.

3. In a medium bowl, stir together the cooled vegetables, ricotta, and salt and pepper to taste.

4. Preheat the oven to 350°F. Set out two 9 x 13-inch casserole dishes.

5. Fill each shell with 2 heaping tablespoons of the cheese-and-vegetable filling and arrange the filled shells in a single layer in the casserole dishes. When all the shells are filled, top them with the marinara sauce, sprinkle them with the mozzarella, and bake for 15 minutes, or until the cheese has melted and the sauce is bubbling.

NOTE: Four of these shells are just 292 calories. Pair with a crisp salad and a slice of Garlic Bread (page 56) for a filling, low-calorie meal.

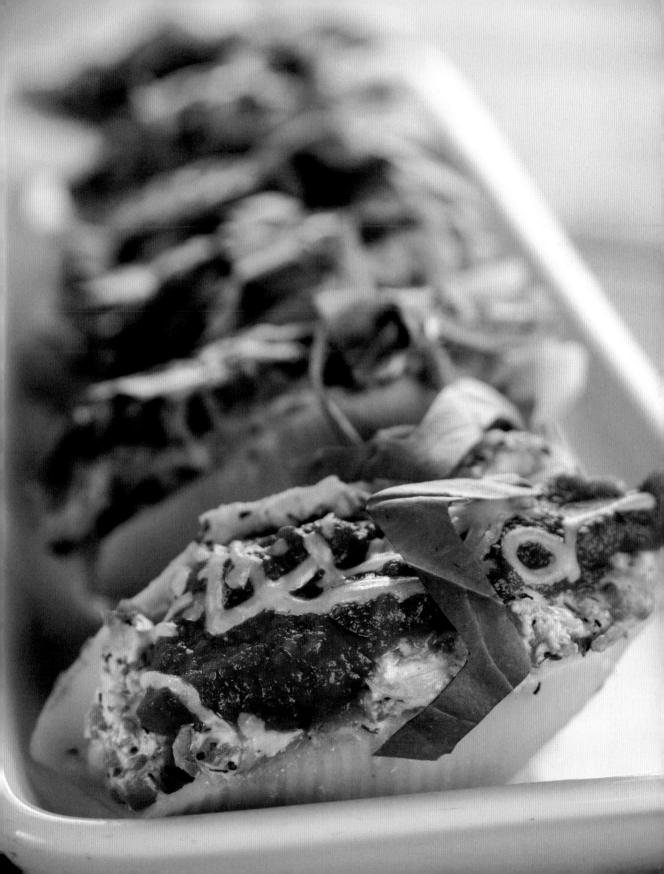

Veggie-Packed Lasagna

Makes 8 servings
Serving size: about 1 cup
Per serving: calories 323; fat 12 g; fiber 8 g; protein 20 g; carbohydrates 40 g

Originally I was going to make this a vegetarian lasagna (which can be easily done—just add ½ cup extra veggies and remove the sausage), but I came across some sweet Italian chicken sausages that inspired me, and that was that. To amp up the veggie component, I chose zucchini and mushrooms—two vegetables that mimic meat—and mixed them with the cooked sausage, and the flavors infused beautifully. This hidden veggie dish is sinfully delicious without the extra fat and calories that leave you feeling guilty and greasy.

If you're not a fan of either mushrooms or zucchini, I implore you to give them another chance. You can't taste the mushrooms at all—they take on all the Italian flavors of the sausage and cook up into the same consistency. If you are allergic, use chopped bell pepper, eggplant, or broccoli florets instead. All are made beyond delicious when covered with tomato sauce and cheese.

1 teaspoon olive oil
1 large onion, finely chopped
⅛ teaspoon kosher salt
3 cloves garlic, chopped
2 sweet Italian chicken or turkey sausages
1 (28-ounce) can diced tomatoes
1 (16-ounce) can tomato sauce
1 (6-ounce) can tomato paste
2 tablespoons Italian seasoning
⅛ teaspoon sugar
2 large zucchini, chopped
2 cups white mushrooms, chopped
¼ cup mascarpone cheese
½ (16-ounce) box no-boil, oven-ready, organic lasagna pasta
1 cup shredded mozzarella cheese

1. In a large saucepan, heat the olive oil over medium heat. Add the onion and salt and sauté until the onion starts to soften, about 5 minutes. Add the garlic and sausages and cook, turning the sausages once, until they are cooked and the onion is transparent, about 10 minutes. (Alternatively, cook everything together in a slow cooker on High; it will take about 1 hour.)

(recipe continues)

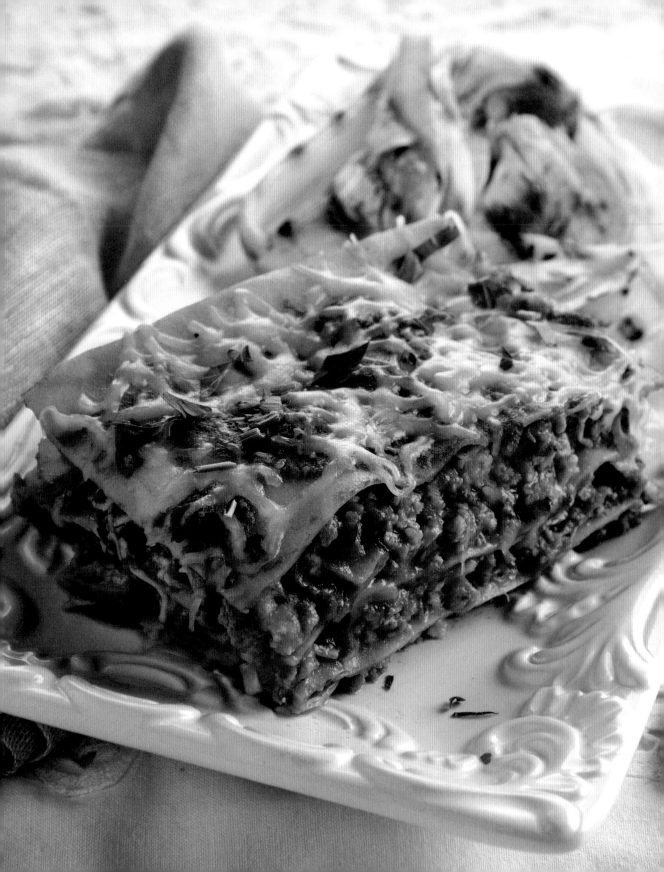

2. Add the diced tomatoes, tomato sauce, tomato paste, Italian seasoning, and sugar and stir to combine. Cover and simmer on low heat for 4 hours. (If using a slow cooker, cook for 6 hours on Low or 4 hours on High.)

3. Remove the cooked sausages from the sauce and transfer them to a cutting board to cool. Chop the sausages and place in a medium bowl. Add the zucchini, mushrooms, and mascarpone to the bowl and fold to combine.

4. Spread about ⅓ cup of the tomato sauce evenly over the bottom of a 9 x 13-inch casserole dish. Top with a layer of uncooked lasagna sheets. Add half the veggie and sausage mixture and spread it out in an even layer, then top with ⅔ cup of the tomato sauce and sprinkle with ¼ cup of the mozzarella. Top the cheese with another layer of pasta sheets, the rest of the veggie and sausage mixture, another ⅔ cup of the sauce, and another ¼

cup of the mozzarella. Add a last layer of pasta sheets and the rest of the sauce. Let the lasagna sit for 20 minutes for the sauce to soak into the pasta sheets.

5. Preheat the oven to 375°F. Place the dish on a baking sheet to catch spillage while baking.

6. Bake the lasagna for 30 minutes. Sprinkle the top with the remaining ½ cup mozzarella and bake for 20 to 30 minutes more, until the cheese has melted and the lasagna is bubbling.

7. Let the lasagna rest for at least 20 minutes; otherwise the slices won't hold together and you will end up with delicious yet unattractive mush. Slice the lasagna in half lengthwise, then slice across three times to make eight squares. Use a small spatula and keep your plates close by—serving lasagna can be a messy affair.

NOTE: It's just as easy to make two trays of lasagna as it is to make one! Simply double the ingredients, then before you bake, cover one tray with foil and move it to the freezer. Defrost in the fridge the morning you want to bake it for a fast and impressive weeknight meal.

That extra tray of lasagna makes a great gift for new parents and hungry college students, too, and won't cost you much at all. Check out your local thrift store for inexpensive glass baking dishes you can give away.

Slow-Cooker Marinara with Meatballs

Makes 8 servings
Serving size: 1 meatball and ½ cup sauce
Per serving: calories 195; fat 8 g; fiber 4.5 g; protein 15 g; carbohydrates 19 g

I'm always shocked to see people wasting money on store-bought, jarred pasta sauce. But what's more shocking to me are the ingredients in it. All those preservatives and other chemicals— how else does "sausage" keep on a store shelf for six months? It baffles me.

I understand that many of the people who buy the jarred sauce are getting it out of convenience, and that's why I created this foolproof slow cooker marinara. I recommend that you make a double batch and freeze the extra so that you have it any time you need it. You can throw this recipe together in the morning, go to work, and come home to the best sauce you've ever had!

Slow-Cooker Marinara
1 large yellow onion, finely chopped
4 cloves garlic, finely chopped
1 tablespoon olive oil
⅛ teaspoon kosher salt
1 (28-ounce) can crushed tomatoes
1 (15-ounce) can tomato sauce
1 (6-ounce) can tomato paste
20 basil leaves, chopped
⅛ teaspoon sugar
Freshly ground black pepper

Meatballs
1 pound lean ground turkey
1 large egg
2 tablespoons freshly grated Parmesan cheese
1 clove garlic, minced
2 tablespoons bread crumbs
1 tablespoon Italian seasoning
½ teaspoon kosher salt
¼ teaspoon freshly ground black pepper

1. Make the marinara: In a slow cooker, mix together the onion, garlic, olive oil, and salt. Cover and cook for 30 minutes on High.

2. Add the crushed tomatoes, tomato sauce, tomato paste, basil, sugar (it helps cut the acid in the tomatoes), and a sprinkling of salt and pepper to taste. Mix well and let it sit on High, covered, while you make the meatballs.

3. Make the meatballs: In a large bowl, combine all the meatball ingredients and mix until just combined (overmixing will make the meatballs tough).

4. With wet hands, divide the mixture into eight portions and roll eight meatballs. Gently drop them into the sauce and spoon the sauce over the meatballs. Cover the slow cooker and cook on High for 4 to 5 hours or on Low for 8 to 10 hours.

Stovetop Directions: In a large saucepan, cook the onion, garlic, olive oil, and salt over medium heat for 15 to 20 minutes, until the onion is soft and transparent. Add the remaining marinara ingredients. Prepare the meatballs as directed, add them to the sauce, cover, and cook over medium-low heat for 4 hours.

A cup of cooked whole wheat pasta is about 175 calories. Together with this recipe, it's about 370 calories per serving, leaving enough calories for a Caesar salad and a slice of 57-calorie Garlic Bread (page 56).

Chapter 9

For the Love of BBQ

Whether you like to barbecue outside or use a grill pan on your stove, you'll love these rich, delicious dishes. I've included lots of chicken recipes to liven up this weeknight staple, plus some fun and delicious ways to make veggies. Don't let the weather stop you—everything in this chapter can be made inside or out.

For stovetop cooking, simply use a grill pan (or griddle if that's all you have) and mimic the instructions. If the BBQ instructions say to cover and cook over medium heat for 10 minutes, simply cover with a lid and cook on the stovetop over medium heat for 10 minutes. These instructions come in handy when you plan on barbecuing and it starts to rain. Just move it inside!

My favorite Smart Swaps for this chapter:

Citrus juice adds flavor and locks in moisture. It tenderizes tough meat and helps caramelize your BBQ dishes without adding sugar.

Whole wheat buns are more nutritious than white buns. You'll stay full longer and will get more fiber and nutrients from unbleached flour.

Olive oil has about the same amount of calories as butter and other oils, but it is more nutritious. If you're going to have oil, you might as well choose the oil that makes you healthier and more beautiful.

Protein-Packed Blue Cheese Buffalo Burgers

Makes 4 burgers
Serving size: 1 burger
Per serving: calories 262; fat 5 g; fiber 2 g; protein 31 g; carbohydrates 20 g

Before you skip over this recipe because it contains buffalo meat, give me one minute of your day to convince you to try this delicious, lean form of protein.

Let's start with the flavor. If buffalo were gross at all, I would just tell you to get lean ground beef. But it tastes exactly like delicious beef, but with more protein, iron, and B$_{12}$ and less fat and calories. Plus it's usually available at your local grocery store. Try this lean and delicious meat yourself. You won't be able to tell the difference, and you'll be doing your body a favor.

1 teaspoon olive oil, for the grill
1 pound all-natural ground buffalo
Kosher salt and freshly ground
    black pepper
½ cup Chunky Blue Cheese Dip (page 108)
4 whole wheat buns
1 cup baby spinach
½ red onion, sliced into thin rings
Spicy brown mustard (optional)

1. Heat a grill to high heat and brush the grill grates with olive oil. (Alternatively, heat a grill pan over high heat and spray it with olive oil.)

2. Make four patties from the meat. Push your thumb into the center and create a little dimple on both sides. This will help the burger cook more evenly and keep a flat patty shape. Gently sprinkle the patties with salt and pepper.

3. Grill the burgers for 7 to 10 minutes, flipping once. Transfer the burgers to a large plate and let them rest for 5 minutes.

4. To assemble the burgers, spread some Chunky Blue Cheese Dip on the bottom of each bun, lay on some spinach and onions, and top with a burger patty. Spread some mustard, if using, on the top buns and place them on the burgers.

NOTE: I love to serve this burger with Asparagus "Fries" (page 171). The combination is only 311 calories, leaving you with enough calories to indulge in a Strawberry Banana Shake (page 236).

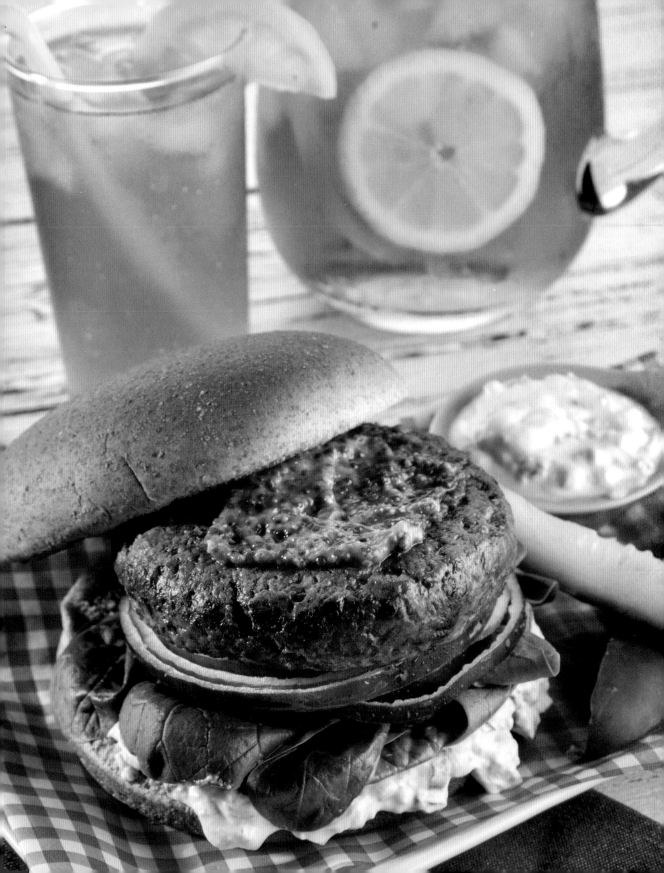

Grilled Chicken "Burger"

Makes 4 chicken burgers
Serving size: 1 chicken burger
Per serving: calories 216; fat 6 g; fiber 2 g; protein 19 g; carbohydrates 19 g

These juicy, flavorful chicken burgers are great for barbecues. They're a good non-beef option for guests, and the leftovers can be used in recipes like the Weeknight Chicken Tacos (page 188) and Chicken, Avocado, and Cheddar Quesadilla (page 94).

This recipe serves four but can easily be doubled and tripled to serve more people.

Chicken Burgers
2 boneless, skinless chicken breasts
1 tablespoon olive oil
Juice of 1 lemon
5 cloves garlic, minced
Kosher salt and freshly ground
    black pepper
4 whole wheat burger buns

Toppings (Optional)
1 tomato, sliced
Caramelized Onions (page 134)
Thinly sliced red onion
Halved romaine lettuce leaves
Ranch Dip (page 105)
Chunky Blue Cheese Dip (page 108)

1. Cut each chicken breast in half horizontally by placing the palm of your hand on the top of a breast and using a sharp, small knife to carefully cut all the way around and through, leaving you with two thin cutlets.

2. Place the chicken in a gallon freezer bag with the olive oil, lemon juice, garlic, and a sprinkling of salt and pepper. Marinate the chicken in the fridge for at least 1 hour or overnight.

3. Heat a grill to medium heat.

4. Grill the chicken for 8 to 12 minutes, flipping once. When the chicken is firm to the touch and cooked through with no pink, it's done.

5. Place a chicken cutlet on each bun. Serve the "burgers" buffet style with all the toppings.

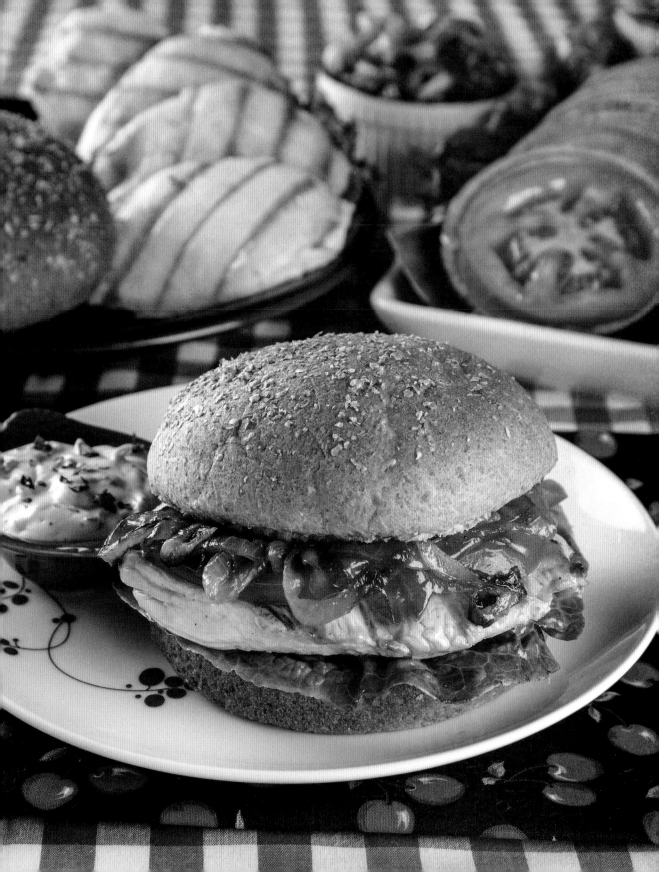

Cheddar-Stuffed Turkey Burgers

Makes 4 turkey burgers
Serving size: 1 turkey burger
Per serving: calories 425; fat 23 g; fiber 4 g; protein 30.5 g; carbohydrates 24 g

I love burgers that ooze cheese when you bite into them, but turkey burgers typically fall apart when you make them with a chunk of cheese in the center. Instead of working against the ingredients, I work with them. If you dice the cheese (rather than shred it), you still get the oozing quality while the cheese also acts to hold the burgers together.

It's important that when you place these burgers on the grill, you don't "play" with them. Don't flip, move, or bother them in any way for the first five minutes or they'll fall apart (this goes for other burgers, too, but especially these). You can also sear them on a hot griddle before moving them to the grill to help them stay together.

1 pound ground turkey
¼ cup sharp cheddar, diced small
2 teaspoons Worcestershire sauce
½ teaspoon kosher salt
½ teaspoon freshly ground black pepper
Olive oil spray
¼ cup Caramelized Onions (page 134)
4 ciabatta rolls or whole wheat buns
4 romaine leaves, halved
1 avocado, sliced
Pickled jalapeños rings (optional)
¼ cup Salsa Ranch Dip (page 105)

1. In a large bowl, combine the ground turkey, cheese, Worcestershire, salt, and pepper. Mix together with your hands until just combined—you don't want tough burgers.

2. Divide the meat mixture into four portions and roll each into a ball. Place each ball on a large plate and squish it down into a flat patty. Press your thumb into the center to create a little well. This will help the burgers keep their flat shape.

3. Spray the grill with olive oil and heat it to medium heat. Grill the patties on direct heat for 5 minutes, covered and undisturbed. Flip once, cover, and grill for another 4 to 6 minutes, until cooked through.

4. To assemble the burgers, smear the caramelized onions on the bottom half of each roll or bun. Top with romaine and place a cooked patty on each. Add avocado slices and jalapeño rings, if using. Smear the top halves of the buns with Salsa Ranch Dip, then place them on the burgers and serve.

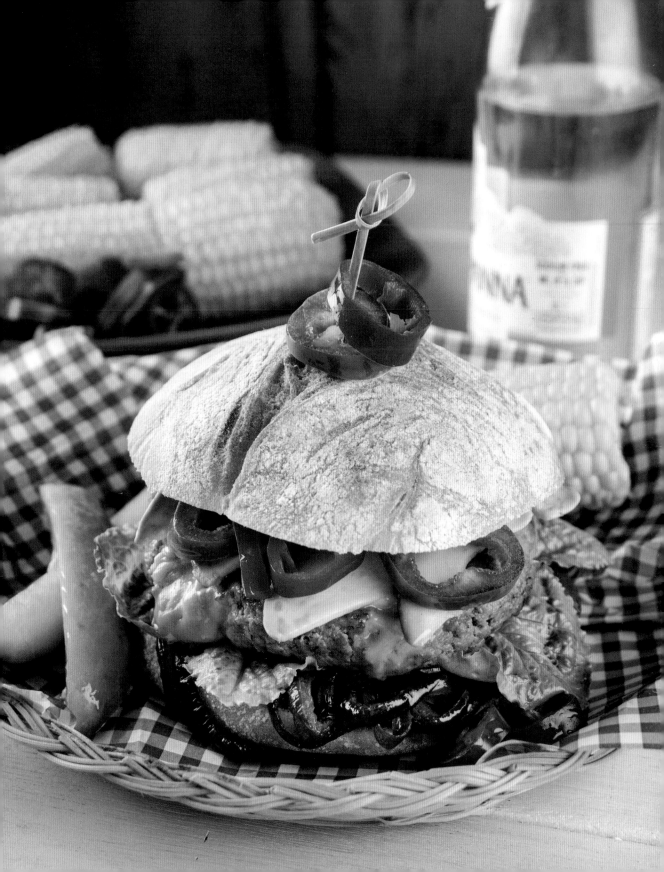

"Everything" Rubbed Steaks

Makes 4 servings
Serving size: 4 ounces
Per serving: calories 178; fat 8 g; fiber 0 g; protein 25 g; carbohydrates 0 g

This recipe was inspired by my time on ABC's The Taste. You can't imagine how intense and exciting it is to be both competing and bonding with great chefs and home cooks on a reality show. The people I worked next to and watched later in the finale inspired and amazed me. And a conversation I had during the taping of the finale left me plotting this recipe all the way home.

During the taping, the remaining three finalists cooked while family members and eliminated contestants watched from bleachers set up onstage. Brad (from Team Anthony Bourdain) and I were trying to figure out what Lee (the Team Bourdain finalist) was making. Brad was betting it was "everything" rubbed steaks. They weren't . . . but I knew they had to be made, and soon!

I love rubs, as they add tons of flavor without adding calories. If you know you're going to freeze the steaks when you bring them home from the store, add the rub first. It really sinks in during the freezing and defrosting stages and makes for easy weeknight BBQ dinners.

1 pound top sirloin steak
4 dashes of Worcestershire sauce
1 teaspoon onion powder
1 teaspoon garlic powder
1½ teaspoons minced fresh chives
1 teaspoon sesame seeds
1 teaspoon kosher salt
½ teaspoon freshly ground black pepper
1 tablespoon olive oil

1. Place the steak on a long sheet of plastic wrap and dash both sides with the Worcestershire sauce. Set the steak aside for 5 minutes to marinate.

2. In a food processor or with a mortar and pestle, grind the onion powder, garlic powder, chives, sesame seeds, salt, and pepper until smooth. Rub half the spice mixture over one side of the steak, flip it over, and repeat on the other side. Tightly cover the steak in plastic wrap, place it on a plate, and refrigerate it for at least 1 hour and up to 24 hours. (If you're freezing it, place the steak in a freezer bag and pop in the freezer.)

3. Remove the steak from the fridge to bring it to room temperature, 20 to 30 minutes before grilling. This will ensure even cooking.

4. Heat a grill to medium heat and brush the grill grates lightly with the olive oil. Place the steak on the grill and close the lid. Grill for 2 to 3 minutes on each side for medium-rare, 4 to 5 minutes for medium, or 7 to 8 minutes for medium-well. Let the steak rest for 10 minutes before slicing into 1-inch strips and serving.

NOTE: For a more impressive dish, cut the 1-pound steak into four equal portions before adding the rub. You'll need to cut the cooking time in half, as smaller steaks will cook faster.

Rum Citrus Chicken

Makes 4 chicken thighs
Serving size: 1 chicken thigh
Per serving: calories 139; fat 6 g; fiber 0.4 g; protein 14 g; carbohydrates 3 g

This is another recipe I start when I get home from the store and freeze for later. Marinating the chicken in the freezer boosts the flavor and makes life much easier, too. Later in the week or month, I can just defrost the chicken in the fridge and move it to the grill for a fast, simple weeknight meal.

This recipe calls for chicken thighs, but the marinade can be used on any cut of chicken, including a whole roasted chicken. If you want to skip the rum, add 2 teaspoons maple syrup in its place.

4 skin-on chicken thighs
Zest and juice of 1 orange
2 cloves garlic, chopped
2 tablespoons dark rum
2 tablespoons chopped fresh cilantro,
  or 1 tablespoon dried
1 tablespoon freshly ground black pepper
1 tablespoon olive oil

1. Place all the ingredients except the olive oil in a gallon freezer bag. Seal the bag and squish the mixture to coat the chicken. Marinate the chicken in the fridge for 1 to 24 hours, or for up to 1 month in your freezer.

2. Heat a grill to medium-high heat and brush the grill grates with the olive oil. Transfer the chicken to a plate and the marinade to a saucepan. Simmer the marinade over medium heat for 5 minutes.

3. Place the chicken skin down on the grill and cook for 10 minutes. Flip the chicken and grill it, dipping the pieces into the pan of marinade once or twice as you go, for 10 to 12 minutes more, or until fully cooked.

4. Set the chicken on a plate to rest for 5 minutes to lock in the flavor, then serve.

Pork Chops in Red Wine BBQ Sauce

Makes 4 pork chops
Serving size: 1 pork chop
Per serving: calories 226; fat 4 g; fiber 0.5 g; protein 40 g; carbohydrates 2 g

Once you make my Homemade Barbecue Sauce, you'll want to spread and slather it on everything, so here's an excuse for you to use it. If you don't have any available, you can use an organic store-bought sauce, but check the ingredients list to be sure there are no preservatives or other chemicals.

I love how the sugars in the barbecue sauce caramelize on these pork chops, making them sweet and savory and all-around delicious. These go great with Veggie Kebabs (page 179) and a side of brown rice, or with the Creamy Mac and Cheese (page 90) and a crisp salad.

¼ cup Homemade Barbecue Sauce
  (see below)
4 pork chops
Kosher salt and freshly ground black pepper

1. Heat a grill to medium-high heat.

2. Lightly coat both sides of the pork chops with barbecue sauce and sprinkle with salt and pepper.

3. Grill the pork chops for 5 to 8 minutes on each side, depending on thickness. Baste with more barbecue sauce as they cook.

4. Let the pork chops rest for 5 minutes before serving.

Homemade Barbecue Sauce

Makes 1 cup

1 teaspoon olive oil
1 shallot, finely chopped
1 clove garlic, finely chopped
⅛ teaspoon kosher salt
1 cup red wine (bold and fruity red wines
  work best, but any red will do)
¼ cup tomato paste
2 tablespoons chili powder
1 tablespoon paprika
1 tablespoon Dijon mustard
1 tablespoon red wine vinegar
1 tablespoon Worcestershire sauce
1 chili in adobo sauce, chopped
1 tablespoon dark brown sugar
½ teaspoon honey
½ teaspoon pure maple syrup

1. In a large saucepan, heat the olive oil over medium heat. Add the shallot, garlic, and salt and cook until the vegetables are soft, about 2 minutes. Add the wine and bring to a simmer, then reduce the heat to medium-low. Cook for 10 to 15 minutes, or until the sauce reduces to about ½ cup.

2. Add the remaining ingredients and 1 cup water. Bring the mixture to a low simmer and cook, stirring often, for 10 minutes. Reduce the heat to low and cook for 45 minutes, stirring often, until the sauce has reduced by a third and thickened (it will continue to thicken as it cools). Let cool completely before refrigerating. The sauce will keep in an airtight container in the fridge for 7 days or in the freezer for up to 3 months.

Asparagus "Fries"

Makes 4 servings
Serving size: about 5 stalks
Per serving: calories 49; fat 3.5 g; fiber 2 g; protein 2 g; carbohydrates 4 g

Next time you're craving salty French fries, try these Asparagus "Fries" instead. You can eat them with your fingers, and they go great with Grilled Chicken Strips (page 176). A fun way to get your kids to eat healthy is to let them eat with their hands.

Try these dipped in Ranch Dip (page 105) or Chunky Blue Cheese Dip (page 108).

2 bunches thick asparagus
1 tablespoon olive oil
1 teaspoon truffle salt, garlic salt,
   or sea salt
½ teaspoon freshly ground black pepper

1. If you have a long fish cooker, grill pan, or square grill press, plan to use that for grilling; otherwise, use wooden skewers, but be sure to soak them in water for an hour to keep them from burning.

2. Heat a grill to medium heat.

3. Snap the tough ends off the asparagus stalks and discard. Place the asparagus in a 9 x 13-inch casserole dish as you go. Add the olive oil, salt, and pepper and toss to coat every stalk.

4. Place the asparagus in the cooker or pan you're using, or if you're using skewers, spear a row of asparagus at the bottom and middle of the stalks, just like a picket fence. This will hold them together and make them easier to flip.

5. Grill the asparagus until they're slightly crispy, about 20 minutes, and serve. These go great over brown rice or alone squirted with lemon juice.

Lemony Drumsticks

Makes 10 drumsticks
Serving size: 2 drumsticks
Per serving: calories 143; fat 9 g; fiber 0 g; protein 14 g; carbohydrates 0.5 g

My daughter loves drumsticks—she calls them "chicken on the bone." I make them often because of their price. Even using all-natural, organic, antibiotic-free drumsticks, you can make this recipe for under eight dollars for a family of five. These are great for kids' parties, football tailgating, and backyard barbecues.

You do need to bake these in the oven for 30 minutes before you move them to the grill, but I promise you'll find them well worth the time. If you're tailgating or camping and don't have access to an oven, get one of those disposable roasting pans and place the chicken in it. Cover and bake right on the grill over medium-high heat for 30 minutes, then move the chicken directly to the grill.

I often place the drumsticks in a freezer bag, add the marinade, and toss the whole thing into the freezer—it takes less than five minutes. Then, when I want to make them for dinner, I defrost them in the fridge in the morning and cook them when I get home after work.

10 chicken drumsticks
Zest and juice of 1 lemon
  (reserve the juiced halves)
4 cloves garlic, chopped
1 teaspoon kosher salt
1 teaspoon freshly ground black pepper
1 sprig fresh rosemary
2 tablespoons olive oil

1. Combine all the ingredients except 1 tablespoon of the olive oil in a gallon freezer bag and marinate in the fridge for at least 1 hour and up to 24 hours—the longer the better.

2. Preheat the oven to 350°F.

3. Dump the contents of the bag into a roasting pan and roast for 30 minutes.

4. Meanwhile, heat a grill to medium heat.

5. Transfer the drumsticks to a large plate and brush them with the reserved 1 tablespoon olive oil. Grill the drumsticks, turning them to avoid burning, until the skin is crispy, 10 to 15 minutes. Transfer the chicken to a platter and serve. Leftovers will keep in an airtight container in the fridge for up to 3 days or in the freezer for up to 4 months.

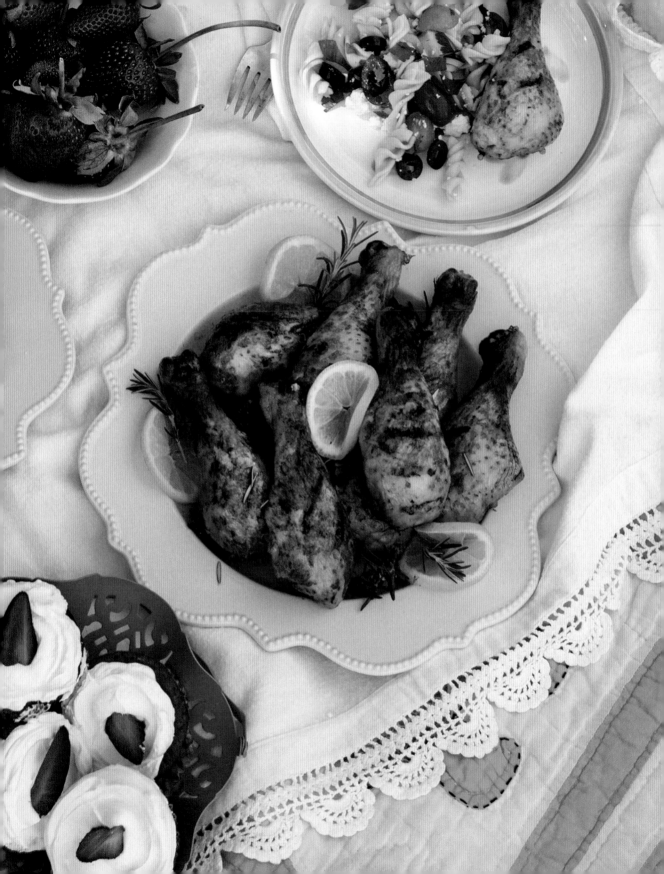

Fajita Chicken Skewers

Makes 4 kebabs
Serving size: 1 kebab
Per serving: calories 50.5; fat 0.5 g; fiber 1 g; protein 7 g; carbohydrates 5 g

This is one of the recipes I hope to eventually be stopped on the street and thanked and hugged for, because I know if I found it in a cookbook, I would do the same!

You can hit the store on your way home, prep, and cook this dish all in under thirty minutes. These chicken skewers are sinfully delicious and full of fat-burning ingredients. Best of all, you get to choose how you want to serve them. I love them in a tortilla with shredded lettuce, Greek yogurt, and an obscene amount of my favorite hot sauce. They're also great atop a salad with my Salsa Ranch Dip (page 105), and leftovers can be chopped to make Chicken Fajita Enchiladas (page 186).

1 onion, cut into bite-size chunks
1 red bell pepper, cut into bite-size chunks
1 chicken breast, cut into ¼-inch-thick
     chunks
2 teaspoons chili powder
1 teaspoon dried oregano
1 teaspoon garlic powder
Olive oil spray
Kosher salt and freshly ground
     black pepper
1 lime, cut into wedges

1. If using wooden skewers, soak them in water for an hour to keep them from burning.

2. Heat a grill to medium-low heat.

3. In a medium bowl, combine the onion, bell pepper, chicken, chili powder, oregano, and garlic powder. Toss to combine.

4. Skewer the ingredients in this order: onion, bell pepper, onion, chicken, bell pepper, onion, chicken, and back to onion again. Keep them close on the skewer and fill the skewer a little more than half full.

5. Spray the skewers with olive oil, sprinkle with salt and pepper, and squeeze a lime wedge over each. (You can prepare the skewers to this stage and let them marinate all day in the fridge for maximum flavor, if you like.)

6. Grill the skewers, turning occasionally, for about 20 minutes, or until the chicken is fully cooked.

7. Serve with tortillas, atop a baked potato, or over chips for homemade fajita nachos.

NOTE: These make great party appetizers; double or triple the recipe for fast and easy crowd-pleasing snacks.

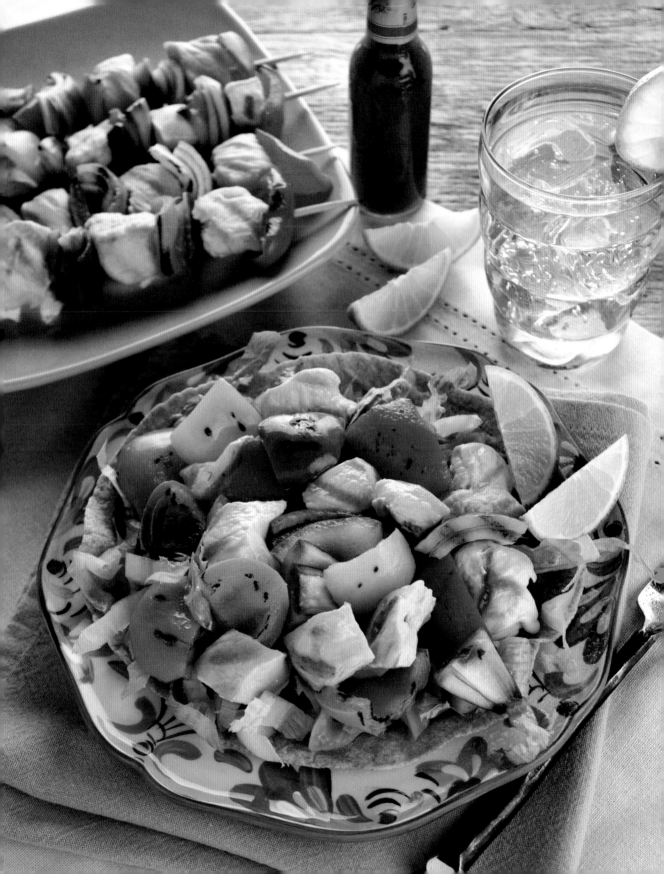

Grilled Chicken Strips

Makes 8 chicken strips
Serving size: 2 chicken strips
Per serving: calories 71; fat 2 g; fiber 0 g; protein 13 g; carbohydrates 0 g

---

Chicken is like a white canvas. If you find it boring, maybe you're using the wrong paint or, in this case, need a good rub, marinade, or sauce. If you make the same recipe over and over, no matter how good the recipe is, you'll get bored. So give your favorite chicken recipe a mini break and try something new.

Between this recipe, the Pesto Chicken Sandwich (page 86), and the Garlic Rosemary Slow-Roasted Whole Chicken (page 220), you'll be taking a new trip with this relatively inexpensive ingredient—one that doesn't end in Boringtown.

I love this chicken in a whole wheat tortilla with my Black Bean Avocado Salad (page 192) or atop a crisp salad—see my Guide to the Perfect Salad (page 18).

2 boneless, skinless chicken breasts
1 tablespoon chili powder
1½ teaspoons garlic powder
1 teaspoon ground cumin
½ teaspoon sea salt
¼ teaspoon freshly ground black pepper
1 teaspoon olive oil

1. Cut the breasts in half lengthwise. Flip onto the cut side and halve again lengthwise so that you get four thick strips from each breast.

2. In a gallon freezer bag, combine all the ingredients except the olive oil. Seal the bag and shake to coat the chicken thoroughly. Marinade the chicken in the fridge for at least 1 hour and up to 24 hours for maximum flavor.

3. Heat a grill to medium heat.

4. Transfer the chicken to a plate and brush each side gently with olive oil. Grill for 5 to 8 minutes on each side, or until cooked through.

5. Set the chicken strips on a fresh plate to rest for 1 to 2 minutes, then serve.

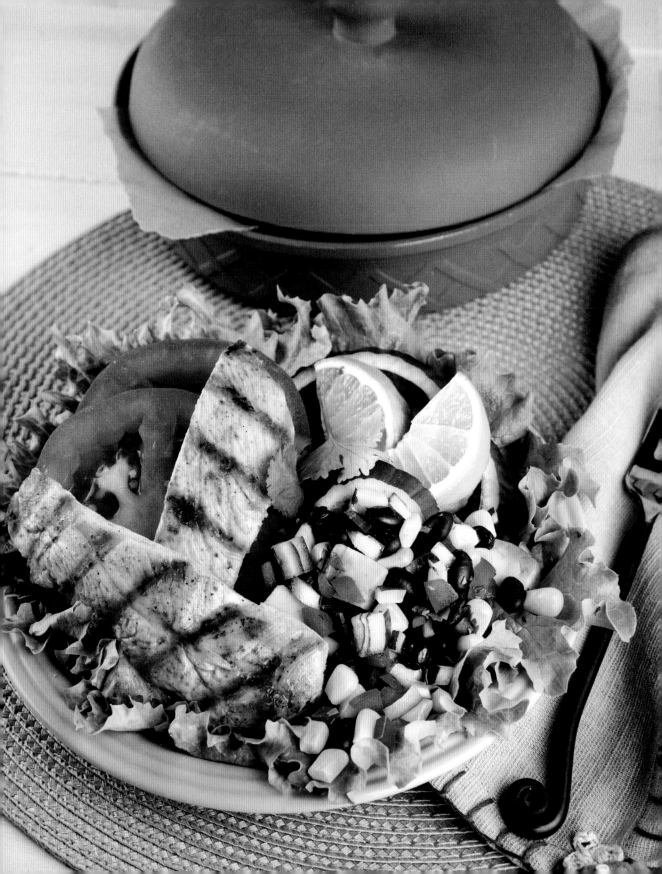

Amusement Park Corn on the Cob

Makes 4 corn on the cob
Serving size: 1 corn on the cob
Per serving: calories 131; fat 8 g; fiber 2 g; protein 2.5 g; carbohydrates 16 g

Amusement park, you ask?

I spent my high school years in Southern California. Just a short drive from my house was an amusement park full of roller coasters, cute boys, and, of course, the very best corn on the cob in the world! This particular amusement park may be famous for its fried chicken, but when I think of that park, it's the corn on the cob that's stayed with me.

I've been trying to replicate the recipe for years, and I think this is pretty darn close. Flavorful and juicy, it's perfect for a backyard barbecue. You can halve the ears of corn for larger gatherings to feed more people and save money.

4 ears of corn, shucked and cleaned
2 tablespoons olive oil
Juice of ½ lime
1 to 2 tablespoons chili powder
(depending on your spice preference)
1 tablespoon garlic salt

1. Heat a grill to medium heat.

2. Rub the corn with the olive oil, place it on the grill, and close the lid. Cook the corn, turning as the kernels start to brown but keeping the lid closed as much as possible, for 10 to 15 minutes.

3. As soon as the corn is done, sprinkle it with lime juice, chili powder, and garlic salt. Serve hot.

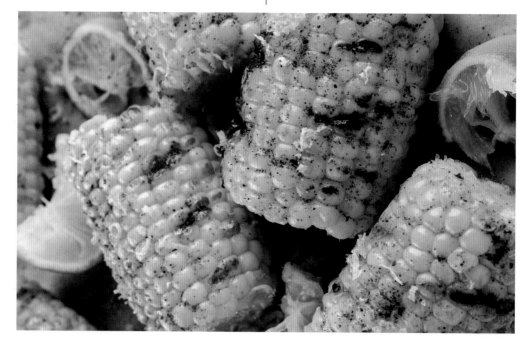

Veggie Kebabs

Makes 4 kebabs
Serving size: 1 kebab
Per serving: calories 70.5; fat 4 g; fiber 2.5 g; protein 2 g; carbohydrates 9 g

I loved kebabs when I was a child. There was something exciting and fun about plucking the vegetables off the sticks. If people in your family don't like veggies, try packaging them in a fun way, such as slain on the plate by wooden swords—it's all in the presentation!

If you're using wooden skewers, to serve kids, cut off the pointy ends with scissors after filling the skewers (or pull the veggies off yourself prior to serving).

1 onion, cut into bite-size chunks
1 bell pepper, cut into bite-size chunks
1 zucchini, cut into ¼-inch slices
1 broccoli crown, cut into florets (leave a little stem for skewering)
2 teaspoons garlic powder
½ teaspoon sea salt
¼ teaspoon freshly ground black pepper
1 tablespoon olive oil
1 lime, halved

1. If you're using wooden skewers, soak them in water for 1 hour before using to avoid burning.

2. Heat a grill to medium-low heat.

3. In a large bowl, combine all the ingredients except the lime and toss until the veggies are coated with spices and oil.

4. Skewer the ingredients in this order: onion, bell pepper, zucchini, broccoli, and back to onion again, working until each skewer is full. Lay the skewers on a plate and squeeze half the lime over them.

5. Grill the skewers directly over the heat, turning occasionally, for about 20 minutes, or until the vegetables are soft and starting to gently char.

6. Transfer the kebabs back to the plate, squeeze more lime juice on top, and serve.

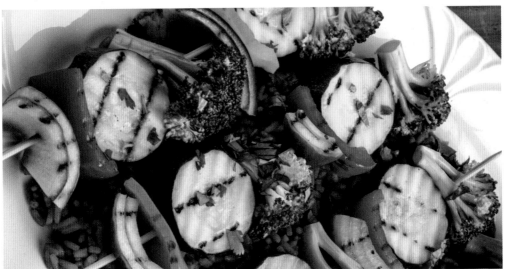

Chapter 10

Mexican Food

Living in California, I get my share of delicious Mexican food, and it would be a shame for you not to have that experience no matter where you live. Here are some of my favorite Mexican recipe makeovers!

Mexican food can easily be made skinny with hidden veggies and delicious with calorie-free spices. Next time you need a spicy kick, try one of these recipes. And don't forget the margarita—I've got you covered with a skinny Watermelon Margarita (page 270).

My favorite Smart Swaps for this chapter:

Greek yogurt tastes just like sour cream, and at only 9 calories per tablespoon, you can have as much as you like.

Lime juice adds a punch of flavor for practically zero calories.

Hidden veggies keep you full and satisfied and increase the serving sizes without increasing the calories.

Chicken Tortilla Soup

Makes 6 servings
Serving size: 1 cup
Per serving: calories 211; fat 8.5 g; fiber 3 g; protein 14.5 g; carbohydrates 20 g

The first time I made this soup, everyone in my family was sick with a cold and I wanted to get them full of good nutrition, so I hit my local farmers' market and got all fresh ingredients. I was also sick, so I made this as simple as possible. Basically, I made fajitas, covered them with water, blended in some tomatoes, and let it boil away.

I loved the ease and method so much that, sick or not, I still make it the same way. So if you're sick, try this ultra-healing soup. It freezes well and can be made in a slow cooker, too, so you can have a bowl of hot, cold-busting Chicken Tortilla Soup whenever you want it.

Soup

1 teaspoon olive oil
1 onion, chopped
1 red bell pepper, chopped
3 cloves garlic, minced
Kosher salt and freshly ground
    black pepper
4 large tomatoes
2 tablespoons chili powder
½ teaspoon ground cumin
1 tablespoon dried oregano
2 jalapeños, seeded and minced (optional)
1 carrot, cut into ½-inch half-moons
1 chicken breast
¼ cup frozen corn

Toppings

1 tortilla
1 teaspoon olive oil
¼ cup 0% Greek yogurt
¼ cup shredded sharp cheddar cheese
⅓ cup chopped fresh cilantro
1 jalapeño, sliced into rings (optional)

1. Make the soup: In a large saucepan over medium heat or in a slow cooker on High, heat the olive oil. Add the onion, bell pepper, and garlic and a pinch of salt and black pepper. Mix to combine. Cover and cook until the onions and bell peppers are soft, about 10 minutes on the stove or 30 minutes in a slow cooker.

2. Place the tomatoes and 1 cup water in a blender and blend into a smooth sauce.

3. Add the chili powder, cumin, and oregano to the pan or slow cooker and cook for 1 to 2 minutes, until you can smell the spices. Add the tomato sauce, jalapeños (if using), carrot, chicken breast, corn, and 1½ cups water. Stir and cover.

4. If you're cooking on the stovetop, bring the soup to a boil over medium heat, then reduce the heat to low and simmer for 30 minutes. If you're using a slow cooker, cook on High for 2 hours or Low for 4 hours.

5. Remove the chicken from the soup and set on a plate. When cool, use two forks to shred the chicken, then add it back to the soup and mix it in.

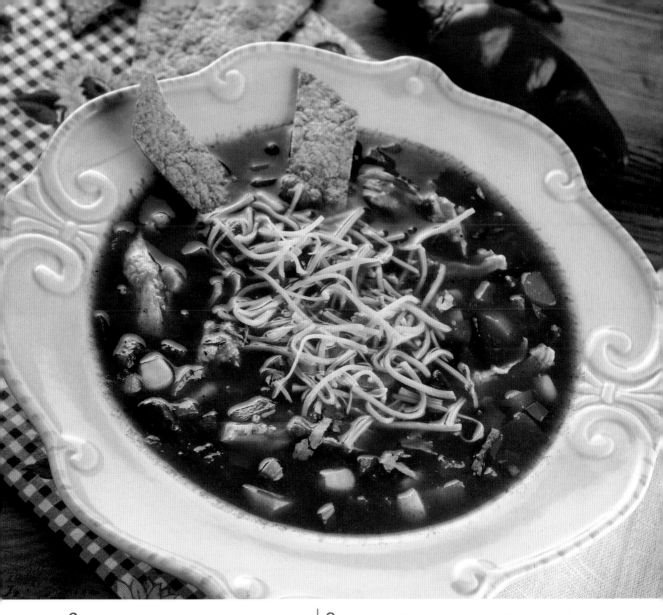

6. Make the toppings: Preheat the oven to 375°F.

7. Brush both sides of the tortilla with the olive oil and cut it into 1-inch strips. Arrange the strips on a baking sheet and bake them for 5 to 8 minutes, or until crispy.

8. To serve, add 1 cup soup to each bowl. For creamy soup, add 1 tablespoon Greek yogurt and mix it in at this time (do not add the yogurt earlier than this). Top with the cheese, tortilla strips, and cilantro. Garnish with jalapeño rings, if using.

> **NOTE:** If you like spice but your family does not, just top your portion of soup with fresh jalapeños. Packed full of vitamin C, they can help you beat a cold, and the spice will help open up a stuffy nose. Just make sure you have tissues handy!

Jalapeño Poppers with Cool Dip

Makes 8 servings
Serving size: 1 jalapeño popper and 3 tablespoons dip
Per serving: calories 52; fat 2.5 g; fiber 0.5 g; protein 3.5 g; carbohydrates 4 g

---

These jalapeño poppers are low calorie and delicious. You can make them mild, medium, or hot. To make them mild, remove all the seeds and ribs (the white membranes). For medium, take out all the seeds and half the membranes, and to make them hot, only remove the seeds.

Jalapeño Poppers
4 large jalapeños
⅛ cup finely shredded sharp cheddar cheese
1 teaspoon garlic powder
2 tablespoons panko bread crumbs
4 tablespoons soft cream cheese

Cool Dip
¼ cup 0% Greek yogurt
2 tablespoons unsweetened almond milk
½ teaspoon garlic powder
¼ teaspoon onion powder
⅛ teaspoon kosher salt
2 tablespoons chopped fresh cilantro
1 sprig fresh dill
1 teaspoon chopped fresh parsley

1. Preheat the oven to 425°F.

2. Cut the jalapeños in half lengthwise and use a paring knife to remove the seeds and ribs.

3. In a small bowl, combine the cheese, garlic powder, and bread crumbs.

4. Lay the jalapeño halves cut side up on a rimmed baking sheet. Spread ½ tablespoon of the cream cheese in each one and top with the cheesy bread crumb mixture.

5. Bake the poppers for 15 minutes, or until the cheese has melted and the bread crumbs are golden brown.

6. For the dip, blend all the ingredients in a blender or food processor until smooth.

7. Serve the poppers with the dip on the side.

NOTE: We love these so much in my house, I make them as a side dish on Taco Tuesday! I get mini sweet bell peppers to make kid-friendly poppers.

You can make the Cool Dip the day before. To store the dip, pour in a plastic container and cover with plastic wrap. Push the plastic wrap over the surface of the dip and push out all the air bubbles. Cover with the lid and store for up to 48 hours in the fridge. I like to use any leftovers as a yummy veggie dip.

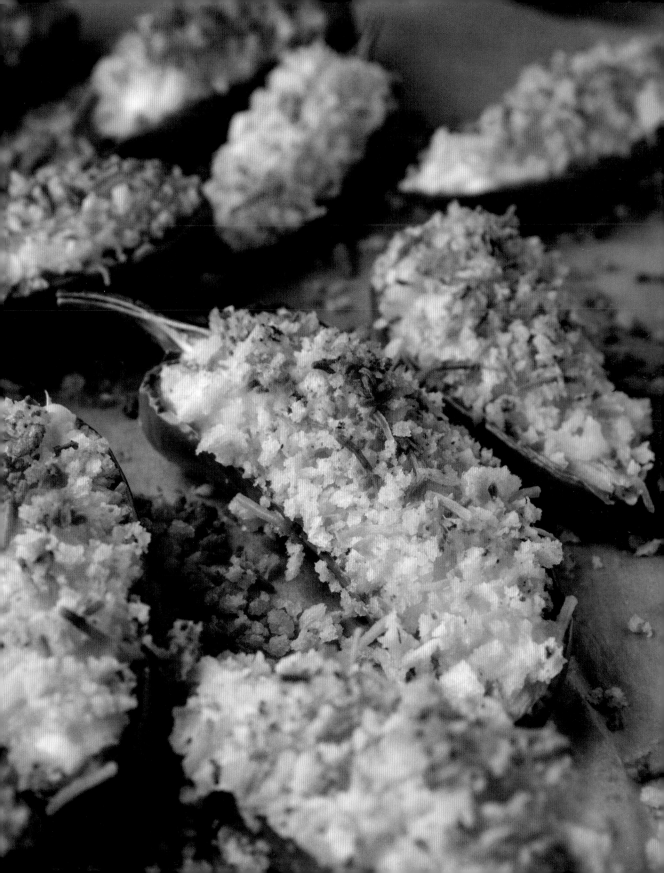

Chicken Fajita Enchiladas

Makes 8 enchiladas
Serving size: 1 enchilada
Per serving: calories 215; fat 7 g; fiber 3.5 g; protein 19.5 g; carbohydrates 19 g

I made these enchiladas one night with left-over Fajita Chicken Skewers (page 174) and it quickly turned into a regular thing. If you end up with extra chicken fajita filling (I always do), save it for a quick lunch. It's great on a baked potato with cheddar and salsa, in a quesadilla, and even with eggs for a delicious breakfast scramble.

These enchiladas freeze beautifully for quick weeknight dinners. Divide them into individual storage containers for microwavable freezer meals. They're quite filling, only 215 calories each, and fantastic with the delicious Black Bean Avocado Salad (page 192).

Chicken Fajita Filling

1 teaspoon olive oil
1 pound chicken breasts, cut into thin strips
1 red bell pepper, thinly sliced
1 onion, thinly sliced
1 jalapeño, seeded and thinly sliced
1 teaspoon cayenne
1 teaspoon chili powder
1 tablespoon dried oregano
1 teaspoon garlic powder
½ teaspoon kosher salt

Sauce

1 jalapeño, seeded and chopped
3 cloves garlic
1 teaspoon fresh thyme leaves
1 onion, chopped
1 (28-ounce) can crushed tomatoes
½ teaspoon ground allspice

Enchiladas

8 corn tortillas
1 teaspoon olive oil
1 cup shredded sharp cheddar cheese
Handful of fresh parsley leaves, chopped

1. Preheat the oven to 400°F.

2. Make the chicken fajita filling: In a large skillet, heat the olive oil over medium-high heat. Add the chicken and brown on both sides until fully cooked, about 5 minutes. Move the chicken to a plate and set aside. In the same skillet, add the bell pepper, onion, jalapeño, cayenne, chili powder, oregano, garlic powder, and salt and cook, stirring often, until the onion and bell pepper are soft, 10 to 15 minutes. Add the chicken (and any juices that spilled out) back in with the vegetables and toss together.

3. Transfer the fajita filling to a plate to cool until you're ready to assemble the enchiladas. Do not wash out the pan.

4. Make the sauce: In the same pan in which you cooked the chicken, combine the jalapeño, garlic, thyme, and onion. Cook over medium heat, stirring, until the onion is soft, about 3 minutes. Transfer the mixture to a blender and add the tomatoes, allspice, and ⅔ cup water. Blend (with the lid slightly ajar) until smooth. Pour the sauce back into the hot pan, bring it to a boil over medium heat, then reduce the heat to low and simmer for 10 minutes.

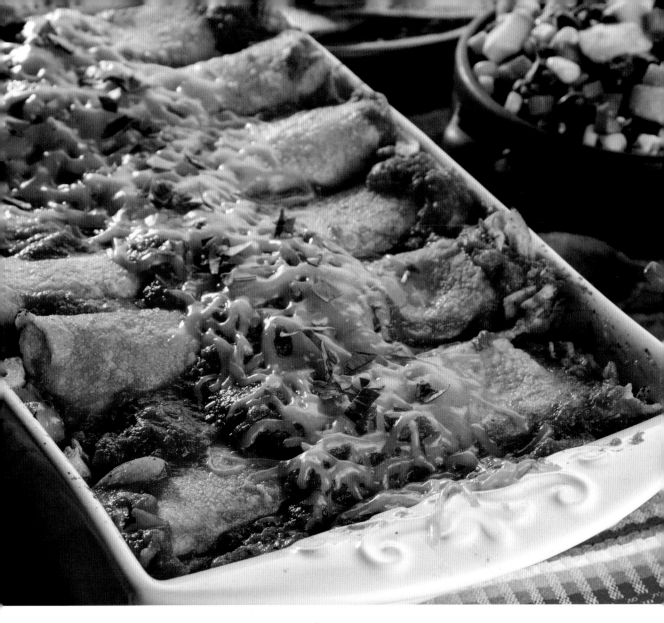

5. To assemble the enchiladas, brush both sides of the tortillas with the olive oil, place them on a baking sheet, and bake for 5 minutes. Set them aside until cool enough to handle.

6. Pour half the sauce on the bottom of a 9 x 13-inch baking dish.

7. Hold a tortilla in your hand and add 1 tablespoon of the cheese and about ⅓ cup of the fajita filling. Roll up the tortilla and place it in the baking dish, seam side down. Proceed to assemble the rest of the enchiladas.

8. Top the enchiladas with the remaining sauce and cheese and bake for 5 minutes, or until hot and bubbling.

9. Garnish the enchiladas with the chopped parsley and serve.

Weeknight Chicken Tacos

Makes 4 tacos
Serving size: 1 taco
Per serving: calories 331; fat 15 g; fiber 6 g; protein 22 g; carbohydrates 28.5 g

Tacos are great for a weeknight meal, but my usual recipe requires too much chopping to whip up quickly. Sure, you can get around all that with some planning, but this recipe gives you a nutritious dinner with five minutes of prep time and fifteen minutes total (faster if you use leftover chicken). Cheaper and better for you than takeout, and just as fast!

Try these on a Tuesday, especially if you have kids . . . they love Taco Tuesday! And if you can get your kids excited about their dinner, getting them to eat healthy is much easier. Serve with some veggie sticks and Salsa Ranch Dip (page 105)—kids love to eat with their hands!

Chicken
2 chicken breasts, or 3 cups diced
    cooked chicken
1 teaspoon olive oil
1 teaspoon fresh lime juice
1 teaspoon chili powder
1 teaspoon garlic powder
Kosher salt and freshly ground
    black pepper

Chunky Avocado Salsa
1 avocado, finely diced
2 tomatoes, finely diced
½ red onion, finely diced
1 teaspoon fresh lime juice
2 tablespoons Five-Minute Salsa
    (page 96; optional, for a spicy kick)
Kosher salt and freshly ground
    black pepper
4 whole wheat tortillas

Toppings
½ cup grated sharp cheddar cheese
1 head romaine lettuce, chopped
¼ cup 0% Greek yogurt (optional)

1. Preheat the oven to 250°F.

2. Coat the chicken in the olive oil (if you have leftover cooked chicken, move to the next step). In a grill pan, cook the chicken over medium-high heat, flipping once, until browned but not cooked through, about 5 minutes on each side. Transfer to a cutting board and chop it into small chunks.

3. Return the chicken to the pan. Add the lime juice, chili powder, garlic powder, salt, and pepper and cook over medium heat for 5 minutes, or until the chicken is fully cooked and blended with the spices.

4. While the chicken cooks, combine all the salsa ingredients in a medium bowl. Taste and adjust the seasonings as desired.

5. Spread the tortillas out on one to two baking sheets. Place in the oven to warm up for 5 minutes. Watch them closely—you just want warm tortillas, not crispy.

6. Put out the warm tortillas, chicken, salsa, and toppings for people to make their own tacos. And there you have it—dinner in 15 minutes!

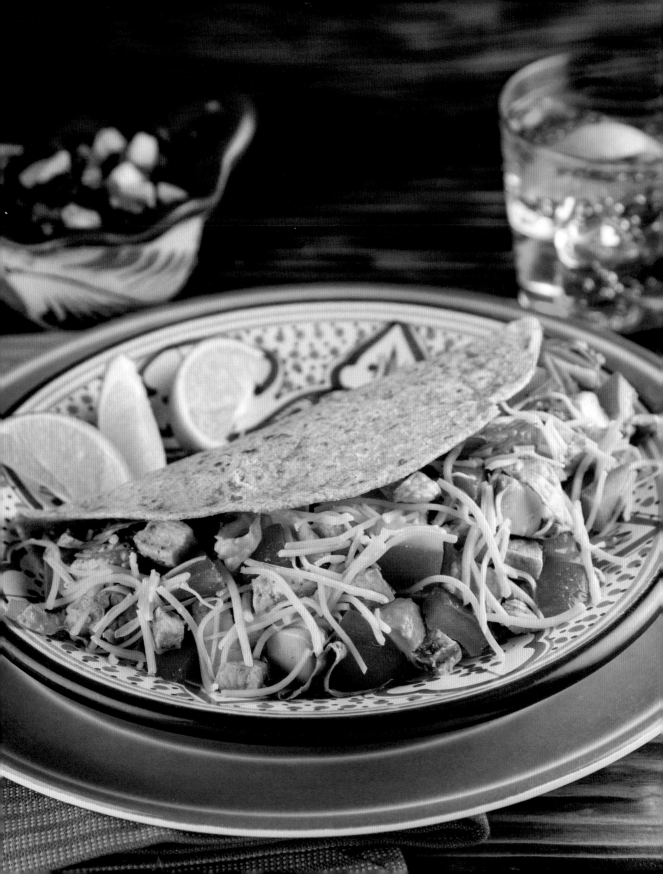

Cilantro Rice

Makes 9 servings
Serving size: ¼ cup
Per serving: calories 88; fat 1 g; fiber 1 g; protein 2 g; carbohydrates 18 g

The only thing better than Spanish rice is Cilantro Rice—fluffy and speckled with green flakes of fresh cilantro. I love it in salads, burritos, and tacos and with all my favorite Mexican main dishes.

Any rice will do, but I highly recommend you go top shelf here and get basmati rice—it has a nice texture, and the price difference between the cheapest and the highest quality is only about a dollar. Yum yum!

¼ cup chopped fresh cilantro, plus more
  as needed
2 green onions, coarsely chopped
1½ cups chicken or vegetable broth
¾ cup basmati rice
1 teaspoon garlic powder
½ teaspoon kosher salt

1. In a blender or food processor, blend the cilantro and green onions with the broth until smooth.

2. In a medium saucepan, combine the broth mixture, rice, garlic powder, and salt. Cover and bring to a boil over medium-high heat. Reduce the heat to low and cook until all the liquid has been absorbed, 15 to 20 minutes. Fluff with a fork and serve.

Spanish Rice: Add 1 cup Five-Minute Salsa (page 96) or your favorite salsa to the saucepan.

Steak Fajitas

Makes 6 servings
Serving size: ½ cup fajitas and 1 tortilla
Per serving: calories 336; fat 7 g; fiber 8 g; protein 25.5 g; carbohydrates 43 g

---

These steak fajitas are easy to prepare on the weekend and cook on a weekday for a fast everyday meal. Store the veggies and steak in a freezer bag with seasonings and freeze along with a packet of tortillas. An hour before you're ready to cook, remove the bag from the freezer and set it on your kitchen counter. Don't worry if the steak is still a little frozen—cooking it while it's still semifrozen will actually keep it from overcooking.

Everyone likes to make their fajitas with their own combination of toppings. and just like you know to taste before you salt, taste before you add high-calorie toppings (grated cheddar adds 114 calories per ¼ cup). Chances are you'll love these with Greek yogurt in place of cheese, and that will save you some serious calories . . . calories you can "spend" on a Watermelon Margarita (page 270).

Steak Fajitas

1 teaspoon cayenne
1 teaspoon chili powder
1 tablespoon dried oregano
1 teaspoon garlic powder
½ teaspoon kosher salt
1 pound sirloin steak, sliced into thin strips against the grain
1 teaspoon olive oil
2 bell peppers, cut into thin strips
2 onions, cut into thin rings
2 jalapeños, seeded and cut into thin strips
1 cup frozen corn
1 (16-ounce) can black beans, drained and rinsed
6 tortillas

Toppings (Optional)

Greek yogurt
Green onions, chopped
Grated sharp cheddar cheese
Five-Minute Salsa (page 96)
Fresh or pickled jalapeños, sliced
Tomatoes, diced
Guacamole Dip (page 104)

1. In a gallon freezer bag, combine the cayenne, chili powder, oregano, garlic powder, salt, and steak. Seal the bag and shake and squish until the meat is well coated in spices. Refrigerate for at least 3 hours and up to 24 hours.

2. In a large skillet, heat the olive oil over medium heat. Add the bell pepper, onion, and jalapeño and sauté until the onion and bell pepper start to soften, about 10 minutes. Add the steak and cook, stirring often, for 5 minutes, until it starts to brown. Add the corn and beans and cook for 3 to 5 minutes, until heated through.

3. Serve with the tortillas and toppings of your choice.

Black Bean Avocado Salad

Makes 6 servings
Serving size: ½ cup
Per serving: calories 131; fat 3 g; fiber 7 g; protein 6 g; carbohydrates 21.5 g

This crisp, salsa-like side dish salad is only 131 calories per serving and as fast to make as opening a can of beans and kicking off your shoes, making it perfect for weeknight meals. In the unlikely event that you have leftovers, try it with chips as a crunchy snack or atop a chicken breast for a simple, protein-packed meal.

1 (16-ounce) can black beans, drained and
    rinsed
1 jalapeño, seeded and minced
1 red bell pepper, diced
½ avocado, diced
½ red onion, diced
¼ cup chopped fresh cilantro
½ cup frozen corn
Juice of 1 lime
1 clove garlic, minced
Kosher salt and freshly ground
    black pepper

1. In a large bowl, combine the beans, jalapeño, bell pepper, avocado, red onion, cilantro, corn, lime juice, and garlic. Gently mix and add salt and black pepper to taste.

2. Marinate at room temperature for 30 minutes to 1 hour and serve.

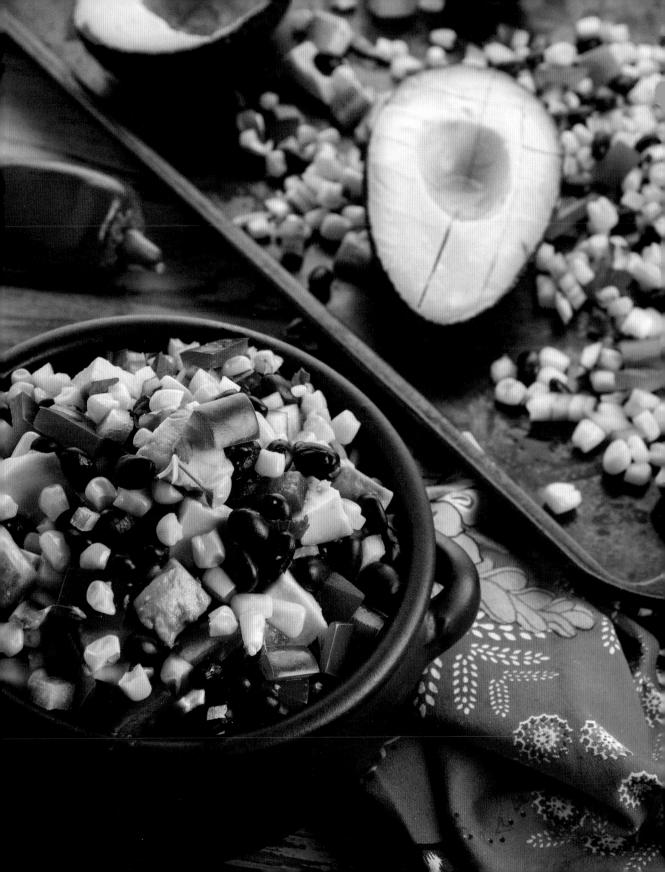

Chapter 11

Comfort Food

Until modern times, we couldn't just walk into a store and buy a steak; we had to hunt and forage. So what happened when food was scarce? Our bodies went into preservation mode, turning food into fat for later. This is why we typically crave fatty foods when we're stressed and under pressure. So next time you crave comfort food, look inward. What's stressing you out? Sit outside and read a book, do a yoga video, or meditate for fifteen minutes. Then go make some of my BBQ Turkey Meat Loaf (page 203) or Skinny Chicken Potpie (page 202) and try to relax. XO.

My favorite Smart Swaps for this chapter:

Hidden veggies are so important here. The BBQ Turkey Meat Loaf, Skinny Chicken Potpie, and Slow-Cooker Pot Roast (page 206) all are more than 50 percent veggies, but they're hidden so well that even the cook forgets how healthy these meals are.

Almond milk gives the Skinny Chicken Potpie an extra creamy sauce and cuts out hundreds of calories.

Loads of spices in these recipes ensure that your taste buds will never be bored! If you think eating healthy tastes boring, try some of these flavorful meals.

Manly Beer Chili in a Slow Cooker

Makes 6 servings
Serving size: about 1 cup
Per serving: calories 301; fat 7.5 g; fiber 10 g; protein 24 g; carbohydrates 37.5 g

Chili is such a crowd-pleaser. Everyone loves it, plus it freezes well and it's easy to make, especially in a slow cooker! I was in the middle of making chili one morning when I opened the fridge to find a premium IPA beer my husband didn't finish the night before. The open beer sat in the fridge, flat and unappealing, but I didn't have the heart to throw it away. So I added it to my chili and this amazing beer chili recipe was born. So the next time you leave a good beer unfinished, don't despair—just freeze it for chili!

I serve this with Easy Tortilla Chips and use leftovers in the Chili Cheese Omelet (page 40) or on a baked potato with some Greek yogurt for a fast lunch.

A very serious note: Do not use light beer, and by light I mean the color. You want a dark beer—IPA, stout, or even a red beer—something with some muscle, or you won't taste it at all and it will just water down your chili. Sad!

Chili
1 teaspoon olive oil
1 pound lean ground turkey
1 large onion, chopped
1 red bell pepper, chopped
2 cloves garlic, chopped
1 jalapeño, seeded and minced
⅛ teaspoon kosher salt
2½ tablespoons chili powder
1 teaspoon ground cumin
2 bay leaves
1 cup really good dark beer
1 (28-ounce) can chopped tomatoes, drained

1 (15-ounce) can black beans, drained and rinsed
1 (15-ounce) can kidney beans, drained and rinsed

Toppings (Optional)
Shredded sharp cheddar cheese
Shredded pepper Jack cheese
Easy Tortilla Chips (page 116)
Green onions, sliced
Five-Minute Salsa (page 96) or your favorite salsa or hot sauce
Greek yogurt (instead of sour cream)
Red onion, chopped
Fresh or pickled jalapeño rings
Tomatoes, chopped
Chopped fresh herbs, such as cilantro, parsley, or basil

1. Preheat a slow cooker on High. Add the olive oil, turkey, onion, bell pepper, garlic, jalapeño, and salt. Cook, breaking the meat up occasionally, until the meat is browned and the vegetables are soft, about 30 minutes.

2. Add the chili powder, cumin, bay leaves, beer, and tomatoes and mix to combine. Cover and cook on High for 4 hours, or turn the heat to Low and cook for 8 to 10 hours.

3. About 30 minutes before serving, add the beans. Crank the heat up to High, uncover, and let the chili bubble away.

4. Remove and discard the bay leaves before serving. If you like, put out toppings for maximum chili personalization. Serve hot!

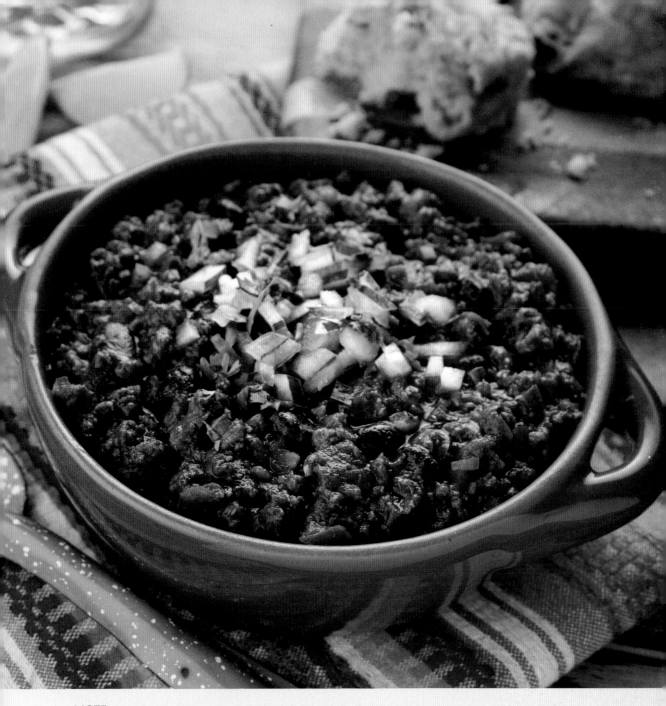

NOTE: You can make this in a large saucepot if you don't have a slow cooker. Brown the meat for 10 minutes instead of 30 minutes. Cover and cook over low heat for 2 hours.

All the alcohol cooks away, so you can feel good about feeding this dish to all ages, but you can skip the beer altogether if you like—this chili is still yummy without it. Replace the beer with ½ cup water for a thinner chili or nothing for thicker chili.

My Mom's Salsa Rice and Chicken Bake

Makes 6 servings
Serving size: ¾ cup
Per serving: calories 182; fat 4.5 g; fiber 2 g; protein 12 g; carbohydrates 22.5 g

My mother had a few signature dishes, and a favorite was a baked salsa rice and chicken. It was a terrific "shove it in the oven" dish for sleepovers. She made it with a well-known boxed "Spanish rice," a product that I now know is full of preservatives and other chemicals that impede weight loss. So I cleaned up the recipe, creating a healthy, all-natural, veggie-filled version that's just as easy as Mom's. I recommend you use leftover chicken in this recipe, and my Five-Minute Salsa goes great in this dish.

Try it yourself for your kid's sleepovers or for an easy no-fuss meal any night of the week. And if you're doing the sleepover thing, check out the Strawberry Banana Shake (page 236) for a fast dessert that won't wire the kids up (it's a sugarless dessert) and that they can make themselves.

¾ cup brown rice
1 yellow onion, chopped
1 red bell pepper, chopped
2 cloves garlic, chopped
1½ cups diced cooked chicken
2 tomatoes, chopped
¼ cup Five-Minute Salsa (page 96)
  or your favorite salsa

1½ teaspoons chili powder
1 tablespoon dried oregano
1 teaspoon ground turmeric
1 teaspoon ground cumin
½ cup shredded sharp cheddar cheese
2 green onions, sliced

1. Preheat the oven to 425°F.

2. In a 9 x 9-inch casserole dish, combine the rice, yellow onion, bell pepper, garlic, chicken, tomatoes, salsa, chili powder, oregano, turmeric, cumin, and 2 cups water. Cover tightly with aluminum foil and place on a rimmed baking sheet to catch any spillage.

3. Bake for 45 to 60 minutes, or until all the water has been absorbed. Heat the broiler. Top the casserole with the cheese and broil for 2 to 5 minutes, until the cheese has melted and is slightly browned.

4. Garnish with the green onions and serve.

NOTE: If you don't have leftover chicken, see the Pesto Chicken Sandwich (page 86) for my easy instructions.

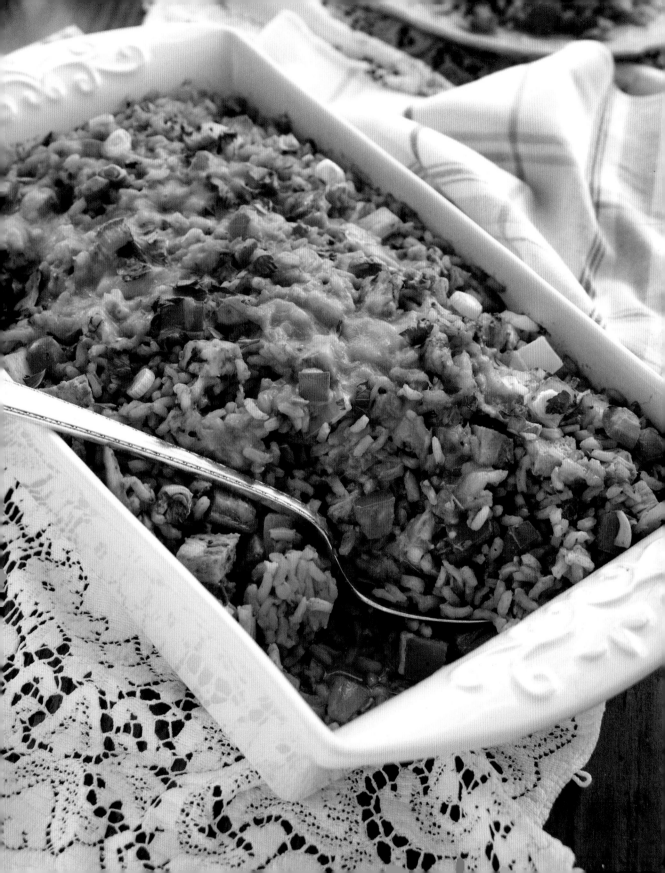

Whole Roasted Chicken with Potatoes and Onions

Makes 8 servings
Serving size: ⅓ cup chicken, skin on (or half a breast, leg and wing, or thigh);
2 potato chunks; and 2 onion chunks
Per serving: calories 414; fat 23 g; fiber 2.5 g; protein 26 g; carbohydrates 22.5 g

This is my family's all-time favorite dinner. I make it for my daughter's birthday every year, and I have no doubt it will be the meal she misses most when she grows up and leaves home.

The chicken is so juicy and delicious, and the potatoes soak up all the chicken drippings and cook down in a delicious rich sauce. I serve it with baked asparagus—you've got the oven on already, so just drizzle 2 bunches of asparagus with 1 tablespoon olive oil, sprinkle with salt and pepper, and toss in the oven on a baking sheet until soft and starting to brown.

This recipe makes for a great dinner party dish. To jazz it up to dinner party status, make a loaf of Garlic Bread (page 56) or Jalapeño Cheddar Scones (page 58) and serve with a crisp salad (see my Guide to the Perfect Salad [page 18]) and either the roasted asparagus (above) or Red and Green Brussels Sprouts (page 228). Make it easy on yourself: ask a guest to bring dessert, or make the Skinny Cheesecake with Raspberry Drizzle (page 238) the day before and you'll really wow your guests!

1 (5-pound) whole chicken
5 medium russet potatoes, quartered
5 onions, peeled and quartered
2 lemons
5 cloves garlic
1 tablespoon spicy mustard (I like Colman's Original English Mustard in this)
1 tablespoon olive oil
10 fresh sage leaves
½ cup white wine (chicken or vegetable stock also works)

1. Remove the top oven rack and preheat the oven to 350°F.

2. Remove the giblets from the chicken cavity and discard or save for another use (like yummy Perfect Chicken Gravy [page 214]). Fold back the wings so the tips don't burn and place the chicken in a roasting pan with the potatoes and onions.

3. To make the marinade, zest the lemons into a small bowl, then use the zester to shred the garlic cloves into the bowl. Stop before the zester gets close enough to cut you and toss the rest of each garlic clove into the chicken cavity. Squeeze the juice from the lemons into the bowl with the garlic and whisk in the mustard and olive oil. Place the lemon hulls in the chicken cavity with 5 sage leaves and truss the legs (tie them together).

4. Drizzle the marinade over the chicken and potatoes. Chop the remaining sage leaves and scatter them over the chicken and potatoes.

5. Roast the chicken, basting three times, for 2 hours, or until browned all over and the internal temperature is 165°F. Transfer the chicken to a cutting board and let it rest for 15 minutes before carving.

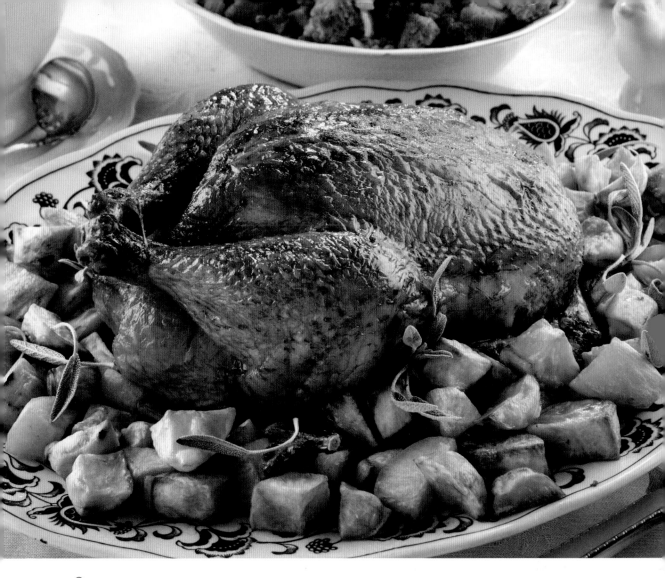

6. Increase the oven temperature to 450°F. Add the wine to the roasting pan and scrape up the brown bits from the bottom of the pan with a wooden spoon. Toss the potatoes and onions with the wine and drippings and roast, stirring occasionally, for 15 to 20 min- utes, or until the pan juices are thickened. Transfer the potatoes and onions to a serving dish and top with any remaining pan juices.

7. Carve the chicken into 8 pieces and serve with the vegetables and pan juices.

NOTE: Chardonnay is my favorite wine with this dish, but any white wine will pair well. Since the dish calls for white wine, get a good bottle (ten to fifteen dollars is a good price point for white wine) and enjoy what's left with your dinner and your guests.

Skinny Chicken Potpie

Makes 6 servings
Serving size: 1 ramekin or 1 cup
Per serving: calories 240; fat 12.4 g; fiber 3 g; protein 5 g; carbohydrates 27.5 g

---

Depriving yourself of your favorite foods only leads to ruin! I love chicken potpie, and if I had to give it up, I would only want it more. So instead of forbidding myself, I created a version that I can enjoy without guilt. To cut calories, I use almond milk and skip the bottom crust—the perfect flaky top crust is enticement enough. Use 4-inch ramekins for a fun individual size or bake the pie in a standard pie pan.

Filling

2 tablespoons unsalted butter
2 tablespoons all-purpose flour
1 onion, finely chopped
½ teaspoon kosher salt
½ teaspoon freshly ground black pepper
2 cups chicken, turkey, or vegetable broth
1 cup unsweetened almond milk
1 cup frozen peas
1 cup chopped carrots
½ cup chopped green beans
1½ cups chopped cooked chicken

Crust

1 cup all-purpose flour
1 teaspoon celery salt
4 tablespoons (½ stick) butter, cold,
   cut into cubes

1. Make the filling: In a large saucepan, melt the butter over medium heat. Add the flour, onion, salt, and pepper and cook until the onion is soft, about 5 minutes. Add the broth and almond milk and cook, stirring often and scraping the bottom of the pan, until the sauce has thickened and coats a wooden spoon, about 15 minutes. Add the peas, car-rots, green beans, and chicken and let the filling bubble away for 5 minutes.

2. Preheat the oven to 425°F.

3. Make the crust: In a medium bowl, combine the crust ingredients. Use a pastry cutter or your hands to work the butter into the flour until it forms pea-size nuggets. Add 3 tablespoons cold water, one at a time, fluff-ing with a fork until the dough starts to pull away from the sides of the bowl. When you grasp it with your fist, it should ball up.

4. Roll out the dough on a clean, floured surface. If you're using ramekins, either use a biscuit cutter or a large cup to cut out tops to fit the ramekins. If you're using a pie plate, roll out the dough into a large circle.

5. If you're using ramekins, set them on a rimmed baking sheet, divide the filling among them, and top with the dough rounds. Pinch the dough over the tops of the ramekins to seal, and poke the center of each with a fork to vent. If you're using a pie plate, set it on a rimmed baking sheet, fill it with the filling, and drape the dough over the top. Pinch along the sides to seal in the filling, and then poke the center three times with a fork to vent.

6. Bake the ramekins for 25 minutes or the pie plate for 35 minutes, or until the crust is golden and the filling is bubbling.

7. Let the potpies cool for a few minutes before serving—they will be hot!

NOTE: This recipe is a great way to use up leftover holiday turkey. You can also swap the chicken for 1½ cups veggies for a vegetarian version.

BBQ Turkey Meat Loaf

Makes 8 servings
Serving size: 1 slice
Per serving: calories 186; fat 8.5 g; fiber 1 g; protein 15 g; carbohydrates 10 g

---

My mother always made meat loaf with barbecue sauce on top and this dish takes me straight back to childhood. A super-tasty sauce like this one adds so much flavor that you can't tell the meat loaf is almost 50 percent veggies. I serve this with Garlic Roasted Potatoes (page 226) and a crunchy salad (see my Guide to the Perfect Salad on, page 18).

2 teaspoons olive oil
1 onion, finely chopped
1 red bell pepper, finely chopped
3 cloves garlic, minced
1 pound ground turkey
2 large eggs
½ cup grated Parmesan or Pecorino Romano cheese, or a mixture
¾ cup bread crumbs (page 81)
1 tablespoon Worcestershire sauce
1 tablespoon balsamic vinegar
2 tablespoons Italian seasoning
1 teaspoon kosher salt
½ teaspoon freshly ground black pepper
½ cup Homemade Barbecue Sauce (page 170)

1. Preheat the oven to 350°F. Spread 1 teaspoon of the olive oil in a loaf pan and place the pan on a rimmed baking sheet. If you don't have a loaf pan, oil a rimmed baking sheet.

2. In a large skillet, heat the remaining 1 teaspoon olive oil over medium high heat. Add the onion and bell pepper and sauté for 5 to 10 minutes, until soft. Add the garlic and sauté, taking care that it doesn't burn, for 1 to 2 minutes, or until soft. Remove the veggies to a plate to cool.

3. In a large bowl, add the cooled onion mixture and the remaining ingredients except for ¼ cup of the BBQ sauce. Mix with your hands until just combined (overmixing will make a tough meat loaf).

4. Transfer the meat mixture to the loaf pan and shape it into a loaf. (If you don't have a loaf pan, just mold the meat loaf into an oval on a rimmed baking sheet.) Top with the remaining BBQ sauce.

5. Bake for 60 minutes, or until the internal temperature is 165°F. Let the meat loaf rest for 10 minutes, then cut it into eight slices and serve.

NOTE: Meat loaf sandwiches are a legendary leftover meal! Save a few slices and sandwich them between whole wheat bread, tomato slices, romaine lettuce, and cheddar cheese. Serve with Ranch Dip (page 105) with veggie sticks for a fast dinner or filling lunch.

Crispy Pan-Fried Pork Chops

Makes 4 pork chops
Serving size: 1 pork chop
Per serving: calories 314; fat 12.5 g; fiber 0 g; protein 44 g; carbohydrates 4 g

Sometimes you just need a fried pork chop . . . it's the truth! That's when I crave these amazing pork chops, adapted from a delicious Nigella Lawson fried lamb chop recipe and made skinny by cutting down on the oil. A delicious crisp salad with homemade dressing is perfect with this rich dish; see my Guide to the Perfect Salad (page 18) for ideas.

Use a good-quality, fresh Parmesan cheese here. The dried-up canned kind won't melt, and it won't taste very good, either. Shred the cheese as finely as you can; a little goes a long way.

⅓ cup panko bread crumbs
¼ cup freshly grated Parmesan cheese
2 tablespoons garlic powder
1 teaspoon kosher salt
1 teaspoon freshly ground black pepper
2 egg whites
4 pork chops
2 tablespoons olive oil

1. In a pie tin or shallow bowl, combine the bread crumbs, cheese, garlic powder, salt, and pepper and mix well.

2. In a second pie tin or shallow bowl, gently whisk the egg whites with ½ teaspoon water.

3. One by one, dip the pork chops into the egg whites, covering them completely on both sides and holding them over the bowl to let extra egg drip off. Dunk the chops into the bread crumb mixture, coating them completely and lightly shaking off the excess bread crumbs. Place the chops on a large plate as you finish them.

4. In a large skillet, heat 1½ tablespoons of the olive oil over medium-high heat. Add the chops and cook undisturbed for 5 minutes (or up to 8 minutes for very thick or bone-in chops), until you can see the bottom third of the chops have turned white around the edges.

5. Carefully turn the chops. Add the remaining ½ tablespoon olive oil and gently tip the pan to distribute it under the chops. Cook the chops for 5 to 8 minutes, or until firm to the touch and golden brown, then move them to a paper towel–lined plate to drain before serving.

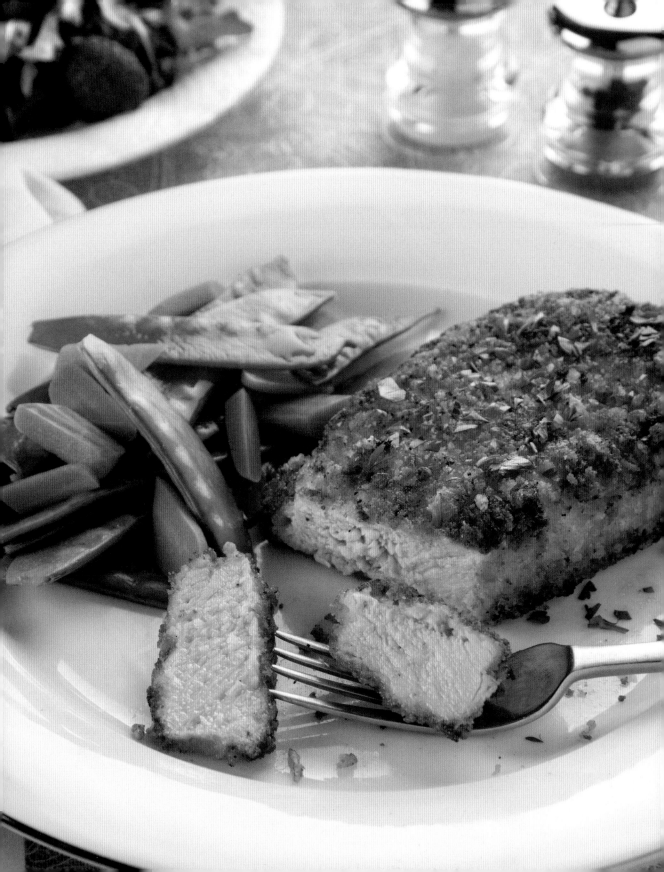

Slow-Cooker Pot Roast

Makes 8 servings
Serving size: 1 cup
Per serving: calories 371; fat 10.5 g; fiber 4 g; protein 44 g; carbohydrates 22 g

This is one of those ultra-comforting meals you'll want to eat next to a roaring fire on a cold, rainy day. It fills your home with the most amazing smells as it cooks all day! Typically pot roast calls for red wine, and I'm not opposed to making it that way, but I've fallen head over heels in love with cooking with beer! I like that I don't have to open a bottle of wine and hope to be in the mood for it later that day—I just pop a bottle of beer, dump it in, and done!

Choose a good, bold beer, ideally an IPA or dark beer. A light beer is a waste of calories; you won't taste it in the dish, so you might as well use water.

1 teaspoon olive oil
Kosher salt and freshly ground
   black pepper
1 (3-pound) chuck roast
2 tablespoons all-purpose flour
2 onions, cut into 2-inch rings
1 (15-ounce) can organic tomato sauce
2 potatoes, halved lengthwise and cut into
   big chunks (see Note)
4 carrots, cut into large chunks
   (about 8 per carrot)
3 stalks celery, cut into large chunks
1 bottle IPA or dark beer
4 fresh herb sprigs (you can use parsley,
   sage, rosemary, thyme, or dried
   bay leaf)
1 teaspoon Worcestershire sauce

1. In a large skillet, heat the olive oil over high heat.

2. Sprinkle salt and pepper all over the roast, then coat it with the flour. Brown the roast on all sides, about 8 minutes, then transfer it to a slow cooker.

3. Reduce the heat under the skillet to medium-high, add the onions, and cook until slightly browned, about 5 minutes. Add the tomato sauce and stir, scraping up any browned bits from the bottom of the skillet. Cook, stirring occasionally, until the sauce reduces and darkens, about 15 minutes.

4. Add the remaining veggies to the slow cooker with the meat.

5. Stir the beer into the tomato sauce and pour the mixture over the vegetables and meat. Add the herbs.

6. Cover the slow cooker and turn it to High. Bring the liquid to a boil over high heat, then decrease the heat to Low to simmer. Cook until the meat is tender and the sauce starts to thicken, about 6 hours.

7. Transfer the roast to a plate to cool slightly. Increase the slow-cooker heat to High and cook, uncovered for 30 minutes, or until the sauce is thickened to your liking. Add the Worcestershire sauce and salt and pepper to taste.

8. Carve the roast into 1/3-inch slices and return them to the slow cooker. Simmer them in the sauce for 10 minutes, then serve the roast with the vegetables on the side.

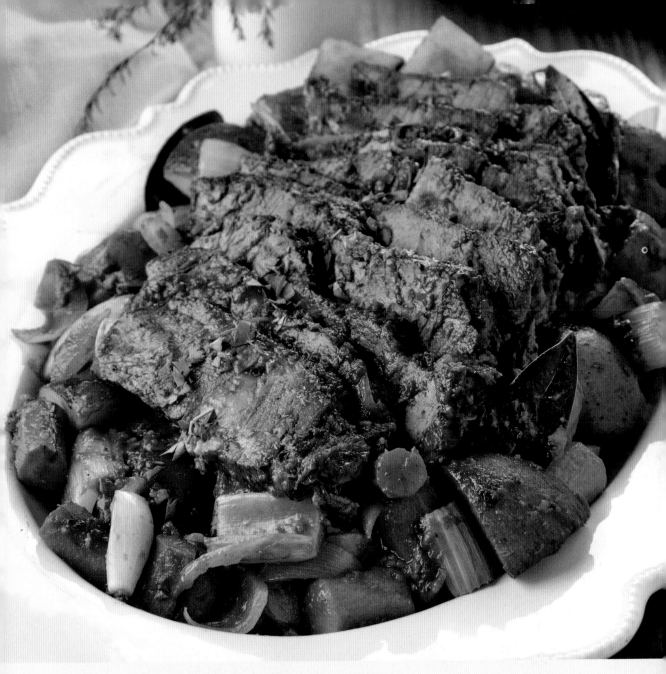

NOTE: The beauty of this dish is in its rusticness. Don't feel like you have to cut all the veggies into perfect shapes. Just make sure all the veggies are about the same size; this way they'll cook at the same rate.

I like to keep the skins on the potatoes, mostly for flavor, but also to cut prep time. I leave this up to you. Peel them if you like . . . or not.

If you don't have a slow cooker, you can do this all in a large pot. Cook on low for 4 hours, covered. When you increase the heat to high to thicken the sauce (step 7), just cook it for 10 minutes.

Overloaded Baked Potatoes

Makes 1 potato
Serving size: 1 potato
Per serving: calories 420; fat 7.5 g; fiber 14 g; protein 28 g; carbohydrates 76.5 g

---

I love recipes that help me use up leftovers, and this is one of them! If you have leftover chicken, save money and time and freeze it for recipes like this one. Or just grill up a chicken breast and shred it (freezing what you don't use). If you're in a rush, you can microwave the potato for 3 to 5 minutes, until soft.

I filled this delicious, filling, and ultra-guilty-tasting meal with metabolism-boosting ingredients like bell pepper, onion, beans, and yogurt and age-defying ingredients like olive oil and avocado. This tastes like a guilty pleasure, but acts like a spa treatment for your body!

Serve half a potato as a great side dish with the Tomato Basil Mozzarella Panini (page 66) or a whole potato on its own as a filling lunch or quick dinner.

1 medium russet potato
½ teaspoon olive oil
1 red bell pepper, coarsely chopped
½ red onion, chopped
1 clove garlic, minced
2 tablespoons canned black beans, drained and rinsed
2 tablespoons frozen corn
¼ cup shredded cooked chicken (skip this for a vegetarian meal)
¼ cup 0% Greek yogurt
¼ avocado, diced
1 teaspoon hot sauce (optional)
1½ teaspoons chopped fresh cilantro

1. Preheat the oven to 350°F.

2. Wash the potato and stab it with a fork a couple of times on each side. Bake right on the oven rack for 60 minutes.

3. Meanwhile, in a medium skillet, heat the olive oil over medium heat. Add the bell pepper, onion, and garlic and cook, stirring often, until the pepper softens, about 10 minutes. Turn the heat to low and add the beans, corn, and chicken. Cook for 2 minutes to warm everything up.

4. Place the potato in a bowl. Slice open the top and squeeze the ends to open the potato. Top with the chicken mixture, yogurt, avocado, hot sauce (if using), and cilantro and enjoy.

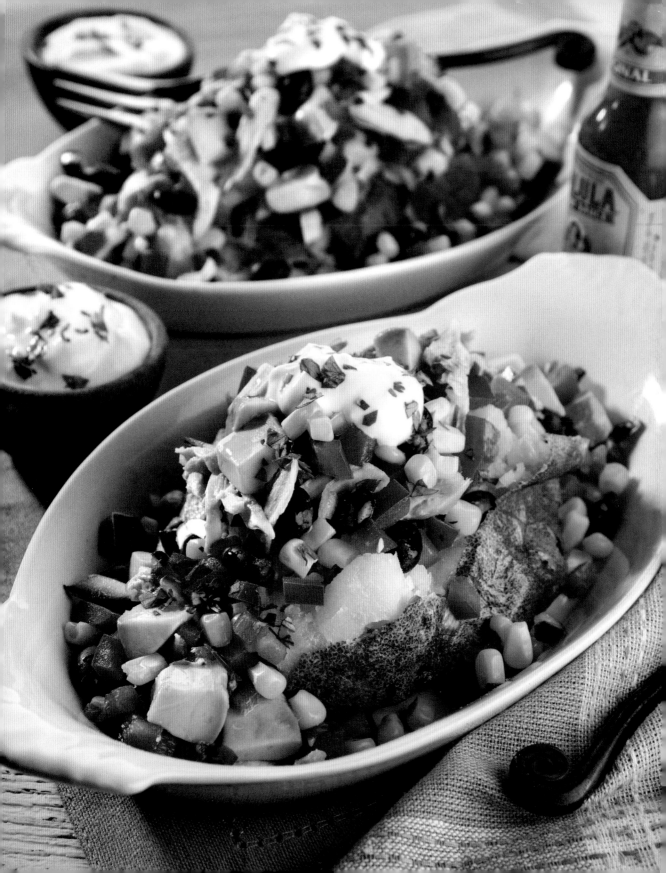

• *Chapter 12* •

Let's Celebrate

I still remember the first holiday dinner I hosted—everyone arrived and the turkey was still frozen. Oh, the nightmare! I remember standing at the sink, pouring water into the cavity, begging the darned bird to defrost already. My skills have improved since then, and I wanted to give you some recipes that take the guesswork out of the holidays while helping to keep your dietary goals in sight. (For starters, brine that turkey!) I include money-, time-, and calorie-saving tips to help you keep your sanity during the holidays and keep the focus where it belongs—on your family.

My favorite Smart Swaps for this chapter:

Maple syrup has one-third fewer calories than sugar and honey, plus it has a great rich flavor that adds complexity to any dish.

Garlic is a staple in all my cooking. Not only is it extremely good for you, but it adds tons of flavor without adding calories!

Almond milk is just 60 calories per cup, a far cry from the 150 calories per cup for whole milk. Just be sure to get unsweetened.

Flawless Brined and Roasted Turkey

Makes 1 turkey
Serving size: 4 ounces
Per dark meat serving: calories 183; fat 5 g; fiber 0 g; protein 33 g; carbohydrates 0 g
Per white meat serving: calories 158; fat 1 g; fiber 0 g; protein 34 g; carbohydrates 0 g

I still have nightmares about my first turkey. Let's just say it didn't go as planned, and it took me years to find the courage to try again. Eventually I realized that roasting a turkey can be quite easy—but roasting a brined turkey is almost foolproof.

If your turkey is still partially frozen, no big deal—the brine will thaw it. Worried about a dry turkey? Don't fret; the brine locks in the moisture! Do you tend to forget to baste the turkey? No problem! You can get by with basting it just twice! Honestly, once you brine a turkey you'll never go back—you'll wake up early on holiday mornings and see that cooler in the middle of your kitchen and smile.

Brine

1 cup kosher salt
1 tablespoon whole black peppercorns
1½ teaspoons allspice berries
    (these look like colorful peppercorns!)
1½ teaspoons ground ginger
1 cinnamon stick
¼ cup pure maple syrup
1 carrot, sliced
1 stalk celery, halved
1 green onion, halved lengthwise

Turkey

1 fresh or frozen turkey, any size
2 tablespoons olive oil

Aromatics

1 cinnamon stick
1 apple, cored and sliced
1 onion, peeled and quartered
4 sprigs rosemary
10 sage leaves
2 sprigs thyme
4 cloves garlic

Equipment

Plastic cooler large enough to hold the
    turkey
Kitchen twine
Oven-safe meat thermometer

1. Two to three days before you roast the turkey, remove it from the freezer and defrost it in the refrigerator. (If you forget to do this, don't fret; just add less ice to the cooler later in the directions.)

2. The day before you roast the turkey, brine it. Ideally you want the turkey to sit in the brine for 12 hours. Start the brine in the morning to allow time for it to cool.

3. To a large stockpot, add 1 gallon water and all the brine ingredients. Bring to a boil over medium-high heat and stir until the salt is dissolved. Let the brine cool to room temperature, then transfer the pot to the refrigerator. Refrigerate until very cold, at least 4 hours.

4. Remove the giblets from the turkey cavity and reserve them to make Perfect Turkey Gravy (page 214). Place the turkey in the cooler, breast side down, pour the cool brine with all the veggies and peppercorns over the turkey, and pour in 1 gallon of heavily iced water (see Note). If the turkey isn't covered by water, add more until it is. Brine the turkey overnight for 12 to 16 hours, flipping it once.

5. Remove the top rack in your oven and move the bottom rack to the lowest setting. Preheat the oven to 450°F.

6. Remove the turkey from the brine and rinse it well with cold water, inside and out. Discard the brine. Place the turkey in a roasting pan and pat it dry with paper towels.

7. In a microwave-safe bowl, combine all the aromatics with 1 cup water. Microwave on high for 5 minutes and carefully, with oven mitts on, dump the mixture into the turkey cavity. Fold back the wings and truss the legs together with kitchen twine.

8. Rub the olive oil all over the turkey, insert the thermometer into the thickest part of the breast (without hitting bone), and roast the turkey for 30 minutes. Lower the oven temperature to 325°F and cook according to the list below, basting the turkey every hour. However, be aware that oven temperatures may vary, which will affect cooking times.

Total cooking times, including the first 30 minutes:

8- to 12-pound turkey: about 2 hours

13- to 16-pound turkey: about 3 hours

17- to 20-pound turkey: about 4 hours

21- to 25-pound turkey: about 5 hours

9. Cover the turkey with aluminum foil if it starts to burn. When the internal temperature hits 165°F, carefully transfer the turkey to a carving board. Do not discard the drippings; you'll need them to make gravy.

10. Let the turkey rest for 20 minutes to lock in the juices and ensure a deliciously juicy turkey dinner. Carve and serve.

NOTE: If the turkey is frozen and it's too late to defrost in time for the meal, use less ice in the heavily iced water (about half and half), as the turkey itself is a big ice cube. Check the turkey every 4 hours to make sure it doesn't thaw too fast and spoil; add more ice to keep it frigid. This method is not ideal, just for emergency situations.

Perfect Turkey or Chicken Gravy

Makes 6 cups
Serving size: ¼ cup
Per serving: calories 17; fat 1 g; fiber 0 g; protein 0.5 g; carbohydrates 1 g

---

I'm putting a strict ban on jarred or canned gravy. If you're making a roasted turkey or chicken dinner, you have everything you need to make gravy on hand already, and your home-made version will have fewer calories and zero preservatives. When you clean your turkey or chicken, just be sure to keep the giblets; they are needed for this recipe. Hey, you paid for them already—you might as well use them!

The quantities are all based on making enough gravy for a turkey dinner, but obviously you won't need as much gravy for a 5-pound chicken as a 20-pound turkey. For chicken gravy, change the quantity of chicken broth to just 2 cups, and start cooking the gravy earlier than the chicken as this recipe takes 2½ to 3 hours to make.

1 teaspoon olive oil
1 onion, thinly sliced
Giblets from your turkey or chicken
    (discard the liver)
Kosher salt
8 cups (2 quarts) turkey or chicken broth
    (less if making a smaller bird—see
    headnote)
1 bay leaf
3 sprigs fresh herbs (parsley, sage,
    rosemary, or thyme—whatever you're
    using in the turkey or chicken recipe)
Drippings from the turkey or chicken
2 tablespoons all-purpose flour
1 teaspoon Worcestershire sauce
Freshly ground black pepper

1. While the turkey is roasting or before roasting the chicken, in a large saucepan over medium-high heat, combine the olive oil, onion, giblets, and a pinch of salt and cook until the neck is browned, about 15 minutes. Add the broth, bay leaf, and herbs. Bring to a boil, cover, and lower the heat to a simmer. Cook for 2 hours.

2. Carefully filter the broth through a mesh sieve into another large saucepan. Let the solids cool a bit, then discard. Simmer the strained broth on low heat.

3. When the chicken or turkey is done, transfer it to a cutting board to rest. Pour the juices from the roasting pan into a large degreasing cup. Add ½ cup of the hot broth to the roasting pan and scrape the brown bits from the pan with a wooden spoon. Add the liquid and brown bits to the degreasing cup.

4. In a large saucepan, heat 2 tablespoons of the fat from the top of the degreasing cup over medium heat. Whisk in the flour and cook the roux, whisking until a paste forms and browns, about 10 minutes.

5. Gradually ladle all the hot broth into the roux, whisking as you go to avoid lumps. Add the drippings from the degreasing cup, minus the fat, and cook, stirring often, until thick, about 10 minutes. Add the Worcestershire sauce and salt and pepper to taste. Serve hot or store for up to 1 week in your fridge or up to 1 month in your freezer.

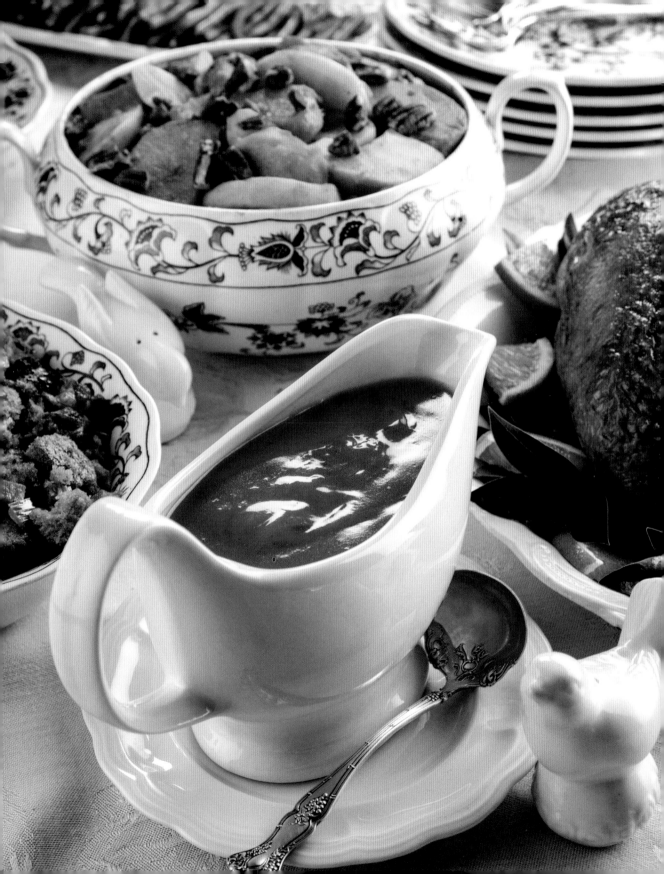

Creamy Mashed Potatoes

Makes 6 servings
Serving size: ½ cup
Per serving: calories 134; fat 2.5 g; fiber 2 g; protein 5 g; carbohydrates 23 g

It's surprisingly easy to cut calories from mashed potatoes, so if you're attached to your grandmother's hundred-year-old recipe, just incorporate my Smart Swaps, because nothing beats an heirloom recipe! In this dish I replace the butter with a little Gruyère cheese and some of the potato water. I also add some garlic salt (or powder) to give it a kick of flavor, use almond milk in place of heavy cream, and add a little Greek yogurt to make it oh-so-creamy.

The flavor of these potatoes intensifies if you keep them overnight in the pan in the fridge before baking, which is also convenient for holiday cooking! But you won't have any complaints if you serve these mashed potatoes immediately. This recipe can easily be made to yield 12 or 18 servings by doubling or tripling the ingredients.

2 teaspoons garlic salt (or garlic powder
    with a pinch of salt)
4 medium russet potatoes
½ cup unsweetened almond milk
3 tablespoons grated Gruyère cheese
3 tablespoons 0% Greek yogurt
Kosher salt and freshly ground
    black pepper

1. Fill a saucepan two-thirds full with water, add 1 teaspoon of the garlic salt, and set it next to your cutting board.

2. Peel the potatoes and cut them into large chunks, placing them in the water as you go to keep them from browning. Bring the potatoes to a boil over medium-high heat for 15 to 25 minutes, or until they almost fall apart when you stick them with a fork.

3. Drain the potatoes, reserving ½ cup of the potato water in a bowl. Add the remaining 1 teaspoon garlic salt, almond milk, and cheese to the pan with the potatoes.

4. Use a potato masher to smash the potatoes to your desired consistency, adding potato water as needed.

5. Add the yogurt and salt and pepper to taste. If you're not serving the mashed potatoes right away, transfer them to a casserole dish, cover with plastic wrap, and refrigerate. To reheat, remove the wrap and bake at 350°F (or whatever temperature your oven is set to) for about 20 minutes, or until warmed through.

Cherry-Glazed Ham

Makes 30 servings
Serving size: 4 ounces
Per serving: calories 275; fat 14 g; fiber 0 g; protein 34 g; carbohydrates 2 g

---

Have you seen the price of HoneyBaked Ham? It's shocking! They're delicious hams, but I just can't bring myself to spend fifty dollars when I can get an uncooked ham on sale for as low as ten dollars. I set out to beat the beloved Honey-Baked Ham, and I believe I have. My mother-in-law is such a HoneyBaked Ham disciple that she sends them as gifts. I made this dish one Easter, and she called a week later for my recipe. I knew then that it was a triumph.

Let's talk about ginger ale. Don't buy diet; you need the sugar in regular ginger ale so that the ham gets a nice crust (and anyway, diet sodas are filled with chemicals that have been proven to cause weight gain). Also, get the best-quality ginger ale you can find! I go for ginger beer, which doesn't contain alcohol—it's just ginger ale made with as much care and celebration as a microbrew beer. Hansen's makes a nice all-natural ginger ale that's sold in most grocery stores if you have a hard time finding ginger beer or top-shelf ginger ale.

Ham gives you endless possibilities for leftovers, so I make a 10-pound ham for my family of three and we enjoy it for days and weeks! The key is portioning out and freezing the leftover ham to suit your needs. Use these leftovers in the Overloaded Baked Potatoes (page 208) or for yummy sandwiches and pasta bakes.

Ham
1 (10-pound) uncooked ham
1 onion, quartered
2 cloves garlic
1 tablespoon whole mixed peppercorns
2 bottles good ginger ale or ginger beer

Cherry Glaze
3 tablespoons all-natural cherry jam
   (don't get sugar-free)
½ teaspoon dark rum (optional)
1 teaspoon paprika
½ teaspoon ground ginger

1. Make the ham: Rinse the ham well with cold water, then submerge it in a big bowl of cold water for 1 hour to remove excess salt (this will also help tenderize it).

2. Preheat the oven to 350°F.

3. In a large roasting pan, place the ham, onion, garlic, and peppercorns. Pour the ginger ale over the ham and cover the roasting pan with foil. Roast for 4 hours. Set the ham aside to cool slightly.

4. Increase the heat to 450°F.

5. Make the glaze: In a small pan, combine the glaze ingredients over medium heat and let them bubble up. Turn the heat off and set aside.

6. Cut off and discard the jellylike fat on the ham. Use a very sharp paring knife to cut a diamond pattern into the ham, about ¼ inch into the surface. Spread the prepared glaze over the outside of the ham and roast it, uncovered, for 10 to 15 minutes, or until the outside of the ham is caramelized.

7. Let the ham rest for 10 to 15 minutes, then use a sharp knife to cut it into thick slices and serve.

Roasted Turkey Breast

Makes 10 servings
Serving size: 4 ounces
Per serving: calories 165; fat 2 g; fiber 0 g; protein 34 g; carbohydrates 0 g

My love for turkey is so great that if I could, I would roast one a week! Unfortunately I can't find whole turkeys all year long, but I've found the next best thing: turkey breast. It's easier to cook, baste, and carve than a whole turkey, but it's still impressive and delicious. Try to find a bone-in breast, since the bones impart tons of flavor and keep the meat moist during roasting. I alternate making this recipe and the Whole Roasted Chicken (page 200) for weekly family dinners.

2 sprigs fresh rosemary
2 sprigs fresh thyme
5 fresh sage leaves
4 cloves garlic, chopped
1 (2½-pound) bone-in turkey breast
½ cup chicken broth
1 tablespoon olive oil
1 teaspoon garlic salt
½ teaspoon freshly ground black pepper

1. Preheat the oven to 350°F.

2. Make a bed of the rosemary, thyme, sage, and garlic in the middle of a 9 x 13-inch casserole dish. Place the turkey breast on the herb bed, pour the broth into the dish, and drizzle the olive oil over the turkey skin. Sprinkle the top of the turkey with the garlic salt and pepper.

3. Roast the turkey, basting it three to four times, for 1½ hours. When a meat thermometer inserted into the thickest part of the breast (without touching the bone) reads 165°F, the turkey is done. Let the turkey rest for 15 minutes before carving.

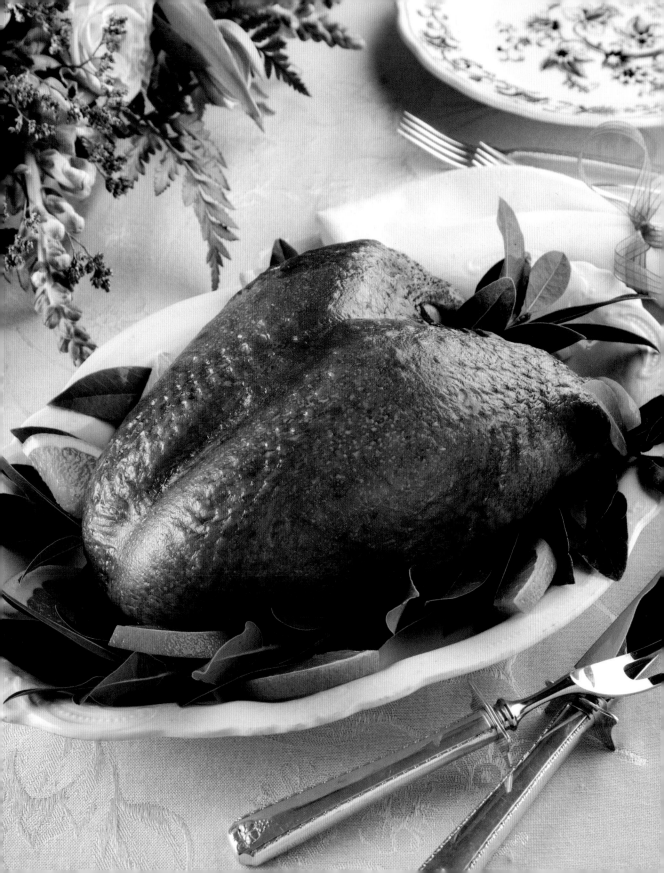

Garlic Rosemary Slow-Roasted Whole Chicken

Makes 8 servings
Serving size: 4 ounces
Per serving: calories 330; fat 25 g; fiber 0 g; protein 23 g; carbohydrates 0 g

Back when I wrote a food column for the local newspaper, my editor asked me for a recipe that would make her boyfriend realize she was wife material. I gave her this recipe, and I'm happy to report that they're happily married!

This chicken is great for a small holiday gathering, a family dinner, or even a quiet date night. It's as easy as it is impressive—even a novice can make a whole roasted chicken! And if folding back the wings, trussing the legs, and shoving the oil mixture under the skin is too much for your first time, then skip the hard stuff: just drizzle over the mixture and stuff the cavity—it will still be delicious.

1 (5-pound) whole chicken
2 tablespoons olive oil
2 large sprigs fresh rosemary
1 head garlic, peeled (you can smash the cloves a bit—they don't need to look perfect)
1 teaspoon kosher salt
1 teaspoon freshly ground black pepper

1. Remove the top oven rack and preheat the oven to 350°F.

2. Place the chicken in a roasting pan. Remove the giblets from the cavity and reserve them to make Perfect Chicken Gravy (page 214) or discard. Fold back the wings so the tips don't burn.

3. In a small food processor or blender, combine 1½ tablespoons of the olive oil, the needles from 1 rosemary sprig, 4 garlic cloves, and the salt and pepper. Blend until smooth.

4. Very gently, push your hand under the chicken's skin, careful not to tear it. Start at the leg cavity and move up to the top of the breasts and then down around the thighs on both sides. Carefully press one-third of the rosemary mixture under the skin of each side of the chicken and gently squish it around to distribute it evenly. Spread the rest of the mixture on the outside of the chicken, then drizzle with the remaining ½ tablespoon olive oil.

5. Chop the remaining garlic cloves in half and place them in the cavity. Fold the remaining rosemary sprig in half and add it to the cavity. Truss the legs together with kitchen twine, if you have it on hand.

6. Roast the chicken, basting three times, for 2 hours. Cover the chicken with aluminum foil if the skin starts to burn. When a meat thermometer inserted in the thickest part of the breast reaches 165°F, it's done roasting.

7. Transfer the chicken to a cutting board and let it rest for 15 minutes. If you take a knife to it too soon, all the lovely juices will spill out and you'll be left with dry chicken. Go distract yourself by making gravy.

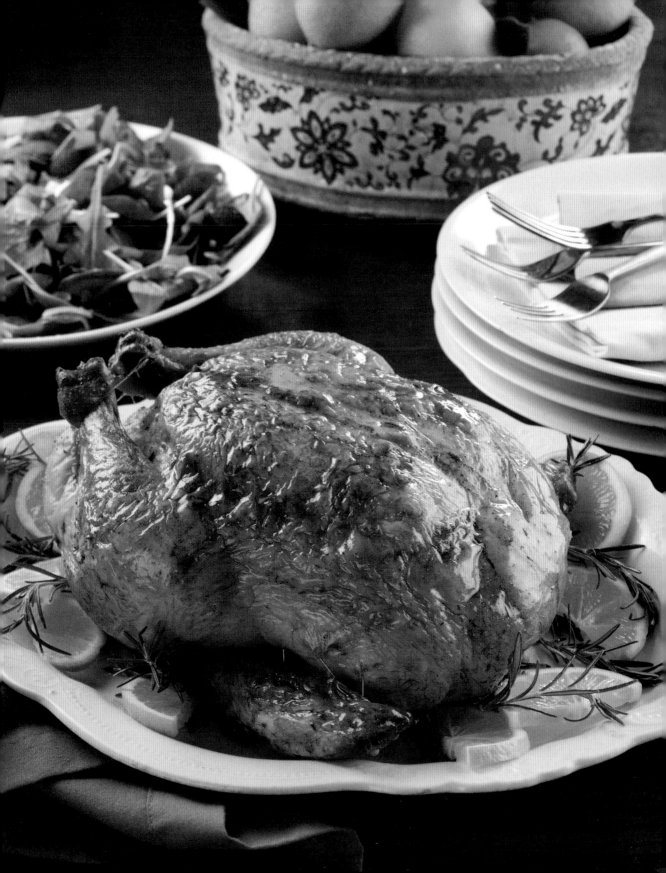

Sausage Stuffing

Makes 15 servings
Serving size: ½ cup
Per serving: calories 130; fat 5 g; fiber 1 g; protein 6 g; carbohydrates 17 g

I love sausage stuffing, but it's usually one of the highest-calorie side dishes on the holiday buffet table, full of fat and carbohydrates with just a touch of vegetables. It's fine once a year, but it's not ideal if you want to enjoy leftovers or avoid the five-pound holiday blues. So what's a girl to do? Get cooking and come up with a healthy, low-calorie, veggie-packed alternative.

I took my favorite recipe, doubled the vegetables, and swapped out the standard white bread for a hearty whole wheat sourdough. This allowed me to drop the quantity of bread, cutting the calories and carbohydrates. I also swapped the sausage from fatty pork to lean chicken or turkey. You're not grilling the sausage and eating it with mustard; you're crumbling it up with loads of other ingredients, so your guests will never miss the higher-fat sausage. (Well, okay, if you're cooking for a world-famous sausage maker, there's a fifty-fifty chance he or she may find you out.)

I bake this the day before a holiday, cover it, and leave it in the fridge. Then all I have to do is heat it up in the oven, saving my sanity on the big day. And if you can find cubed butternut squash, grab it! It will save you time, and you can freeze the rest for later.

1 loaf whole wheat sourdough bread, cut into ½-inch cubes
1 cup cubed butternut squash
2 tablespoons olive oil
1¼ teaspoons kosher salt
¼ teaspoon freshly ground black pepper
1 large onion, chopped
1 bunch celery, including leaves, chopped
2 cloves garlic
2 chicken or turkey sausages
4 cups chicken broth
2 egg whites
1 teaspoon minced fresh thyme
1 tablespoon unsalted butter, cut into tiny cubes

1. Preheat the oven to 375°F.

2. If the bread is not already stale, spread it onto two rimmed baking sheets and toast it in the oven for 15 to 20 minutes, until firm to the touch.

3. In a 9 x 13-inch casserole dish, toss the squash with 1 tablespoon of the olive oil, ¼ teaspoon of the salt, and the pepper. Spread the squash in a single layer and roast it for 35 minutes, or until soft. Remove the dish from the oven and set it aside.

4. In a large pot, heat the remaining 1 tablespoon olive oil over medium heat. Add the onion, celery, garlic, sausages, and 1 teaspoon remaining salt and cook until the veggies are soft and the sausages fully cooked, about 10 minutes. Set the sausages aside on a plate to cool until you can handle them. Remove them from their casings and crumble the meat into the dish with the squash.

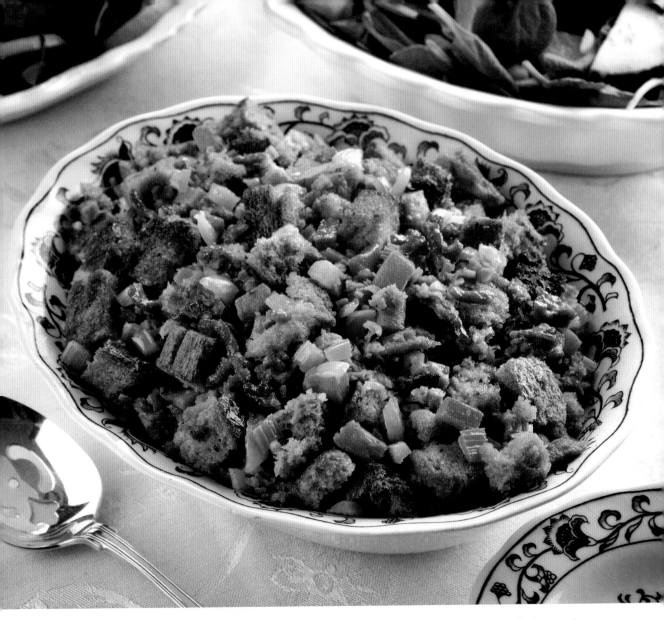

5. Add the broth to the pot with the vegetables and bring to a simmer over medium heat. Turn off the heat.

6. In a large bowl, whisk the egg whites and thyme. Add the bread, squash and sausage mixture, and onion and celery mixture and stir to combine. Transfer the stuffing to the casserole dish. Drop the butter cubes all over the top of the stuffing (this will help it crisp up), then cover with aluminum foil.

7. Bake for 25 minutes, remove the foil, and bake for 20 minutes more, or until the stuffing is crispy and golden in the corners. If you're taking the stuffing to a gathering, bake the first 25 minutes at home and bake the remaining 20 minutes at your destination.

Maple-Glazed Sweet Potatoes

Makes 6 servings
Serving size: ⅓ cup
Per serving: calories 160; fat 5 g; fiber 2 g; protein 1 g; carbohydrates 24 g

I have this obscenely large three-inch blue binder stuffed full of magazine clippings of recipes. Instead of saving cooking magazines, once a year I sit down with a Vanilla Latte (page 268) and go through every single magazine. I pull out recipes I love or want to try and recipes that inspire me. I turn to this binder when I want to make a dish but I'm not quite sure how I want to make it.

When I came home from the farmers' market with some beautiful sweet potatoes, not quite sure how I wanted to cook them, I pulled out my trusty binder and found the full-fat, full-calorie version of this Guy Fieri recipe. I gave it a little calorie makeover and have found that this sweet, flavorful dish is just as satisfying to my guests as the traditional marshmallow-covered version.

Be sure to get sweet apples, not tart—they'll make a better replacement for the marshmallows. I love Gala, Jazz, Honeycrisp, and my personal favorite, Fuji.

3 large sweet potatoes
¼ cup coarsely chopped pecans
1 teaspoon unsalted butter
1½ teaspoons pumpkin pie spice
    (see Note, page 232)
1½ teaspoons chili powder
3 tablespoons pure maple syrup
3 tablespoons dark rum, brandy, or
    whiskey (or the juice of 1 orange plus
    ½ teaspoon chili powder)
1 large sweet apple, peeled, cored, thinly
    sliced, and tossed with a bit of lemon
    juice

1. Preheat the oven to 375°F. Place the sweet potatoes in a 9 x 9-inch casserole dish (no need to pierce them) and bake for 45 minutes, until cooked through. (Feel free to do this when you have turkey, ham, or another dish in the oven to save time.) Set aside the potatoes until they're cool enough to handle. Leave the oven on.

2. In a large skillet, toast the pecans over medium-low heat, stirring often to keep them from burning, for 10 minutes, or until crispy. Add the butter, pumpkin pie spice, chili powder, maple syrup, and rum and bring to a simmer. Cook, stirring often so it doesn't burn, for 10 to 15 minutes, or until thick.

3. Meanwhile, cut off the potato ends and slice lengthwise. Peel off and discard the skins. Cut the potatoes into ¼-inch-thick half-moons.

4. Add the apples and sweet potatoes to the skillet with the spiced pecans, turn off the heat, and toss gently to mix.

5. Transfer the mixture to the casserole dish, drizzling any pan sauces over the top, and bake for 25 minutes, or until the apples and potatoes are super-soft and the dish is bubbling hot. Your kitchen will smell amazing!

NOTE: You can make this dish up to 2 days ahead of time. Cover it with foil, refrigerate, and when you're ready to eat it, just throw it into the oven to heat through.

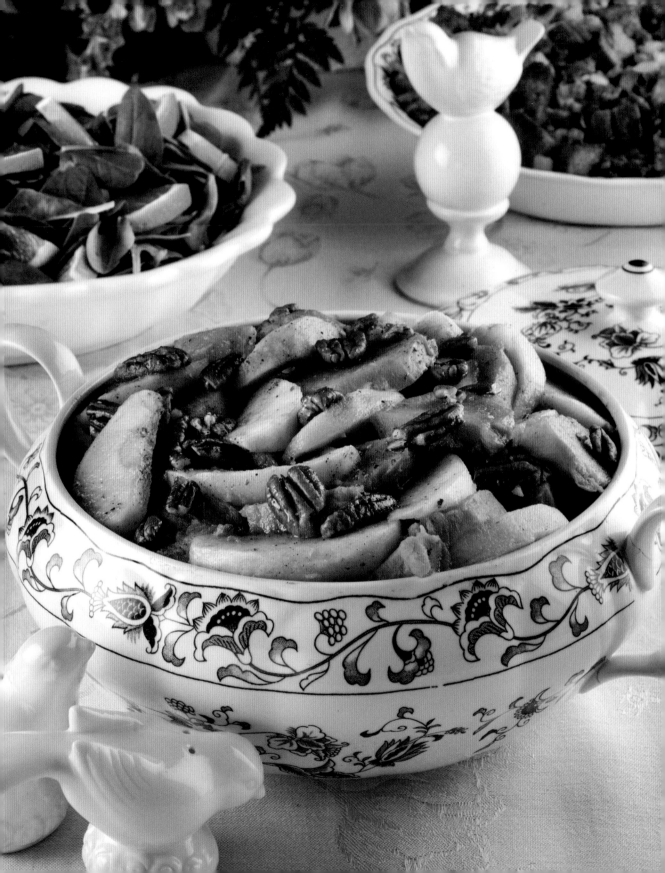

Garlic Roasted Potatoes

Makes 16 servings
Serving size: ¼ cup
Per serving: calories 82; fat 1 g; fiber 2 g; protein 2 g; carbohydrates 16 g

I made similar potatoes while on ABC's The Taste, and everyone loved them! So much so that Chef Ludo Lefebvre told my mentor, Chef Marcus Samuelsson, that he'd made a big mistake by not putting them up as the group dish. We didn't lose, but we didn't win, either, and to this day, I can still hear Ludo's thick French accent commending my crunchy roasted potatoes!

The key to this recipe is the size you cut the potatoes—you want crunch on the outside and a soft center. I've found that 1-inch cubes work great here and cook up quickly, making them fast enough for a weeknight meal but delicious enough for a holiday dinner.

Cloves from 1 garlic head, innermost peels left on
4 large russet potatoes, cut into 1-inch cubes
1 tablespoon olive oil
½ tablespoon unsalted butter, melted
1 teaspoon garlic salt
½ teaspoon freshly ground black pepper

1. Preheat the oven to 350°F.

2. Combine all the ingredients in a large bowl.

3. Tumble the potatoes onto one or two rimmed baking sheets and roast for 10 minutes. Use a spatula to scrape and flip the potatoes over to avoid sticking, then roast for 15 minutes more, or until the potatoes are crispy and golden. Remove and discard the garlic cloves and serve.

NOTE: When I was on *The Taste* I used duck fat in this dish in lieu of olive oil and it was completely amazing, although I believe these are as good (if not better) than the crispy golden potatoes I made on the show. If you have duck fat (or turkey fat during the holidays), use it in this recipe; it adds lots of flavor, and as long as you add only 1 tablespoon in place of the olive oil, you won't be adding any calories.

Nutty Citrus Cranberry Sauce

Makes 6 servings
Serving size: ⅛ cup
Per serving: calories 84; fat 3.5 g; fiber 3.5 g; protein 1 g; carbohydrates 14 g

I know it may be traditional to serve the canned cranberry stuff, but this all-natural version is better tasting and packed with metabolism-boosting ingredients. It goes great on leftover turkey sandwiches and even over Greek yogurt with some Homemade Pumpkin Spice Granola (page 34).

I make this ruby-jeweled sauce a day or two before a holiday gathering. I like it cold or at room temperature, so I get it out of the way, saving stress and time.

3 tangerines
3 cups fresh or frozen cranberries
1 cinnamon stick
1 tablespoon pure maple syrup
2 tablespoons chopped pecans

1. Zest the tangerines into a medium saucepan, then peel and segment the tangerines and add them to the pan. Add the cranberries, cinnamon stick, maple syrup, and 2 tablespoons water.

2. Bring the mixture to a simmer over medium-low heat and cook for 15 minutes, or until most of the cranberries have popped and the sauce thickens.

3. Remove and discard the cinnamon stick, and remove the pan from the heat. When ready to serve, sprinkle the top with the chopped pecans.

Red and Green Brussels Sprouts

Makes 6 servings
Serving size: ⅓ cup
Per serving: calories 64; fat 3 g; fiber 3.5 g; protein 3.5 g; carbohydrates 8.5 g

I love Brussels sprouts, especially when they're covered with Perfect Turkey or Chicken Gravy (page 214), so of course I had to include them in this chapter. They're festive and delicious and low enough in calories that you can go back for seconds and thirds! They're also great on weeknights with Whole Roasted Chicken (page 200) or alongside Creamy Mac and Cheese (page 90). Cook this dish all year round for a healthy side dish you can feel good about serving your family.

30 Brussels sprouts, dark outer leaves removed, halved
1 red bell pepper, cut into small cubes
1 teaspoon olive oil
1 tablespoon shredded Parmesan cheese
1 teaspoon garlic powder
½ teaspoon kosher salt
½ teaspoon freshly ground black pepper
1 tablespoon chopped fresh parsley

1. Preheat the oven to 425°F.

2. Combine all the ingredients except the parsley in a large bowl and mix well.

3. Tumble the mixture onto a rimmed baking sheet and roast for 25 minutes, or until the edges of the Brussels sprouts turn golden brown and the bell peppers soften. Transfer to a serving bowl, sprinkle the parsley on top, and serve.

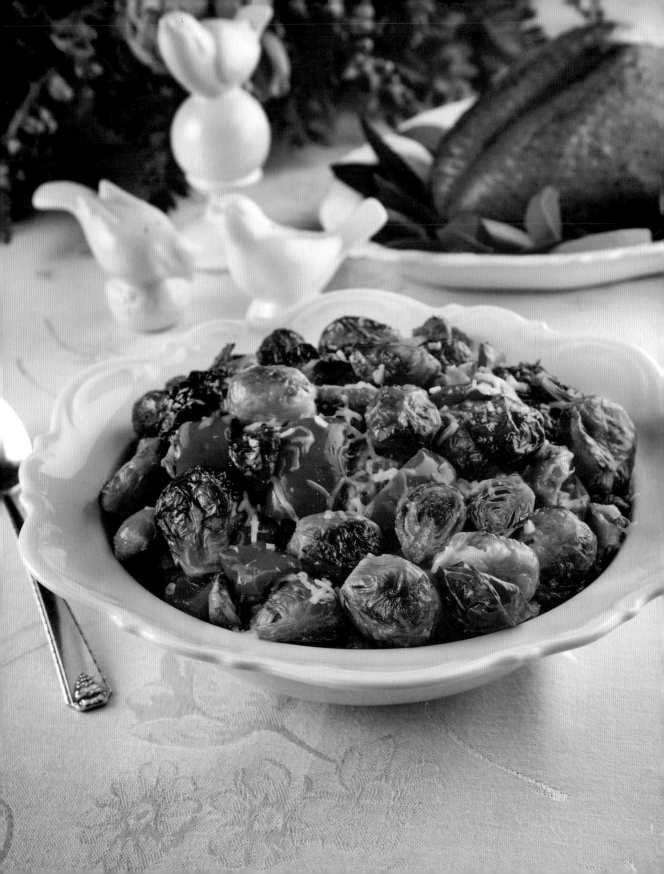

Chapter 13

Sweet Desserts

I often say, "If I had to give up chocolate, I would still be 275 pounds."

I have a sweet tooth that won't quit, and the great thing about the Lose Weight by Eating plan is that I don't have to quit my sweet tooth, either.

In this chapter I give some of the most popular desserts a skinny makeover, shaving hundreds of calories off recipes for desserts like cheesecake and creamy ice pops to make them low in calories and high in nutrition. These sweets that were only occasional treats before have gotten a nip and tuck to turn them into everyday indulgences that are kind to your diet and full of flavor.

My favorite Smart Swaps for this chapter:

Bananas are great in place of ice cream, marshmallows, and butter.

Frozen berries add sweetness to recipes while naturally boosting metabolism.

Greek yogurt can be used in place of heavy cream, ice cream, and butter.

Bananas Foster

Makes 4 servings
Serving size: 3 banana slices
Per serving: calories 93; fat 4.5 g; fiber 1.5 g; protein 2.5 g; carbohydrates 10 g

When it comes to Bananas Foster, cutting calories comes down to reducing the amount of sugar and alcohol. When I tested my skinny version next to a full-sugar recipe, it was so delicious I actually preferred it. The full-sugar version was so overly sweet that my teeth ached; I ran to the bathroom to brush them. But my skinny Bananas Foster was subtly sweet, complex, and elegant. The sauce is a little thicker and more caramel-like than a traditional Bananas Foster sauce, but I prefer it that way.

This dessert is perfect topped with a dollop of homemade whipped cream (page 246) and served with a cup of espresso. Try it yourself tonight!

2 tablespoons unsalted butter
2 tablespoons dark brown sugar
½ teaspoon ground cinnamon
⅛ teaspoon ground nutmeg
    (freshly grated, if you have it)
Kosher salt
3 small bananas, cut in half crosswise,
    then lengthwise
2 tablespoons dark rum

1. In a large sauté pan, combine the butter, sugar, cinnamon, nutmeg, and a pinch of salt. Heat on low until the butter and sugar are melted.

2. Add the banana slices to the pan and spoon the sauce over the tops. Cook for 3 minutes, then flip them over and spoon more sauce on top.

3. When the bananas are soft, another 3 minutes or so, remove the pan from the heat. Add the rum, return the pan to the heat, and use a long lighter or long match to light the sauce on fire. If this is your first time purposely starting a fire in your kitchen, don't stress—it burns out within a few seconds and the flames are very low. Cook this dish on the back burner farthest away from you if you're still nervous.

4. Once the flame burns out, it's time to serve. Divide the bananas into four servings, drizzle the pan sauce on top, and enjoy.

NOTE: If you don't have cinnamon and nutmeg, but you have pumpkin pie spice, you can use it here to save money. It does have ginger in it so the flavor will be slightly different, but it's still super yummy! Use ½ teaspoon pumpkin pie spice in place of the cinnamon and nutmeg.

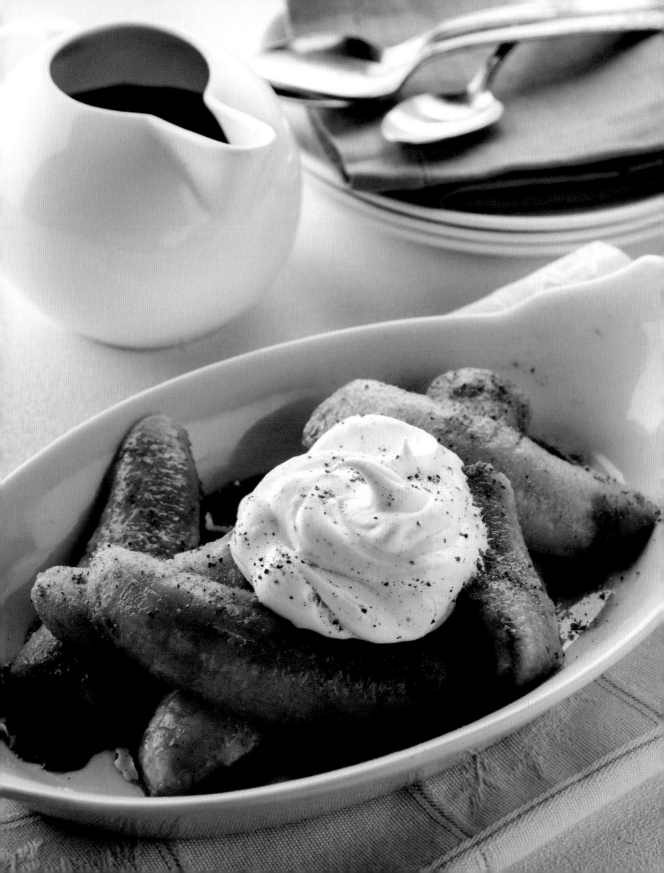

Chocolate, Banana,
and Peanut Butter Blender "Ice Cream"

Makes 6 servings
Serving size: about ⅓ cup
Per serving: calories 124; fat 4 g; fiber 4 g; protein 4 g; carbohydrates 21 g

This recipe is a perfect example of using a Smart Swap; frozen bananas, when blended, have the same consistency as ice cream. So next time your bananas start to freckle, slice and freeze them for use in smoothies in place of ice cream, or defrost and mash them in place of butter in baking recipes, or, best of all, make this blender "ice cream." (I don't have an ice cream maker; I use a twenty-dollar blender I got on sale six years ago, and the "ice cream" still comes out fantastic.)

For those of you looking to break in an ice cream maker with a skinny recipe, don't fret! I'll use my earnings from this book to purchase an ice cream maker, and by my next book perhaps I'll include an ice cream chapter.

4 bananas, cut into bite-size slices and
    frozen for at least 8 hours
1 cup unsweetened almond milk
2 tablespoons unsweetened cocoa powder
2 tablespoons all-natural peanut butter

1. Place all the ingredients in a blender or food processor and blend until smooth.

2. Serve immediately for best consistency and flavor; this "ice cream" won't keep in the freezer.

Almond Joy: Swap almond butter in for the peanut butter and top with toasted almonds and a little flaked coconut.

Nut-Free: Use Greek yogurt in place of the peanut butter for creaminess and a boost of protein.

Freckled: Add 1 tablespoon white or dark chocolate chips or cacao nibs for a freckled crunch.

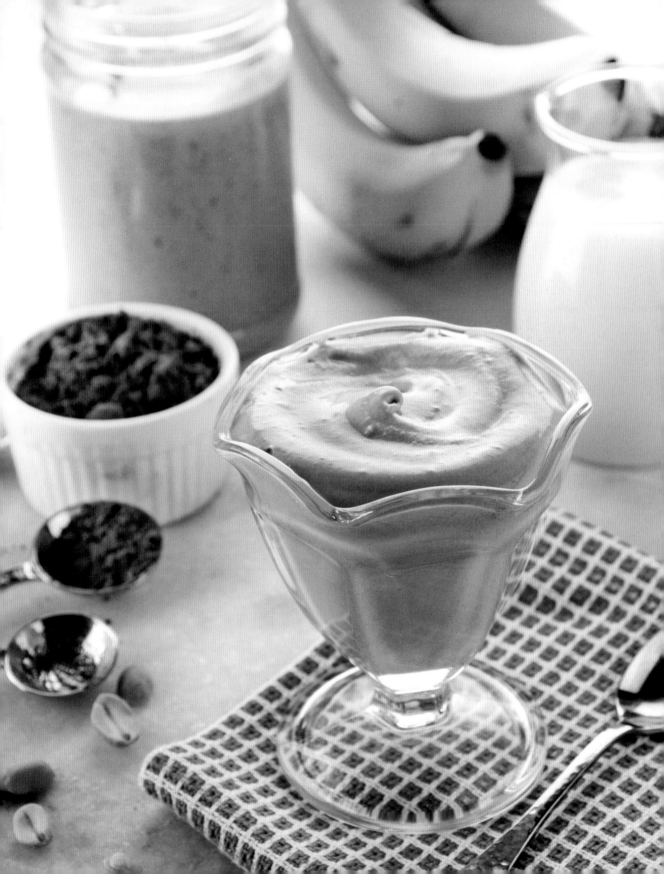

Strawberry Banana Shake

Makes 2 shakes
Serving size: about 2.5 cups
Per serving: calories 137; fat 2 g; fiber 5 g; protein 2 g; carbohydrates 30 g

I love strawberry shakes and I live about a block from an In-N-Out drive-thru, so I made this recipe to keep myself from splurging every time I drove past. I use frozen bananas in place of ice cream to cut more than 900 calories in this recipe makeover.

Keep strawberries in the freezer and you can make this recipe at any time of the year (and save yourself some time). Frozen fruits and vegetables are flash frozen the same day they're harvested, locking in flavor and nutrients, so stock up and enjoy year-round.

1 large banana, cut into bite-size slices and frozen for at least 4 hours or overnight
2 cups frozen strawberries
1 cup unsweetened almond milk
1 teaspoon balsamic vinegar

1. Combine all the ingredients in a blender or food processor. Blend until smooth and serve immediately.

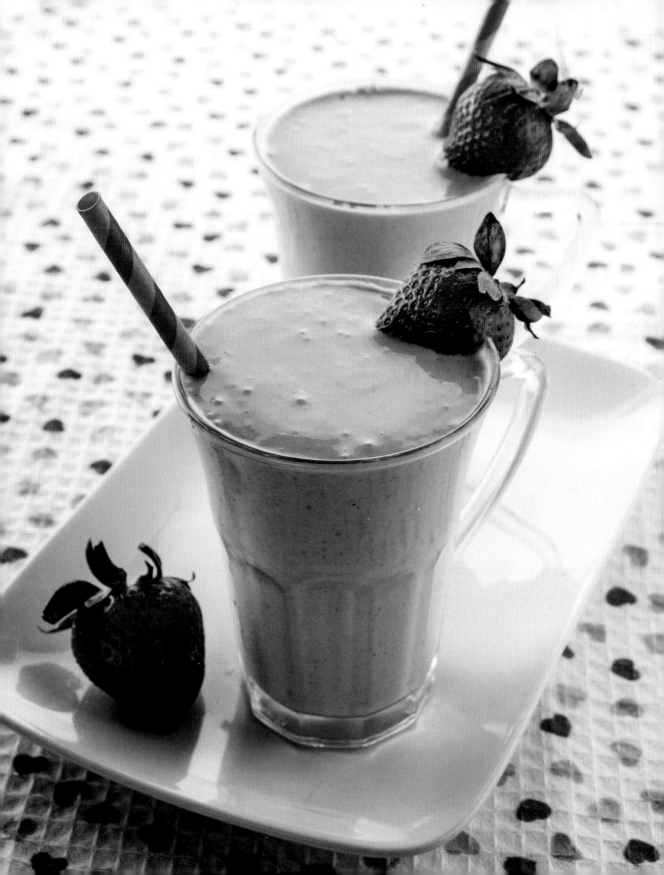

Skinny Cheesecake with Raspberry Drizzle

Makes 16 servings
Serving size: 1 slice
Per serving: calories 137; fat 3 g; fiber 1 g; protein 9 g; carbohydrates 19 g

I think I enjoy decorating this cheesecake almost as much as I enjoy eating it. I summon my inner Jackson Pollock and drizzle and splatter the ruby sauce all over the bright white canvas, sometimes even standing on a stepstool to get the right angle. Creative cooking eases stress, clears my thoughts, and gives me a sense of control, if only for an hour. Give it a shot!

This cheesecake looks beautiful when baked in a round springform pan, but you can just as easily use a 9 x 13-inch glass baking dish lined with parchment paper. And best of all, you won't need a water bath with this recipe. Pick up some organic or all-natural graham crackers at your local health food store or order some online; you don't want any nasty preservatives in this delicious dessert.

Butter wrapper, for the pan

Crust
1 cup crushed graham crackers
2 tablespoons unsalted butter, melted

Cheesecake Filling
3 (8-ounce) packages fat-free cream
   cheese, at room temperature
½ cup powdered sugar
1½ teaspoons pure vanilla extract
¾ cup egg whites
   (from about 4 large eggs)

Raspberry Sauce
1 cup fresh or frozen raspberries
2 tablespoons powdered sugar
½ teaspoon fresh lemon juice

1. Preheat the oven to 350°F. Line the bottom of a springform pan with a circle of parchment paper. Rub a butter wrapper along the inside of the pan to coat the sides. Cut out a large square of foil and wrap it to seal the outside of the pan, securing the bottom and sides. Place the pan on a rimmed baking sheet.

2. In a medium bowl, mix the graham crackers and butter to the consistency of damp sand. (Or use a food processor to crush and combine the crackers and butter, but be sure to wash the processor out before using it for the cheesecake filling.)

3. Dump the crumbs on the bottom of the prepared pan and press them down into a tightly packed and even layer.

4. Bake the crust for 10 minutes, then set it aside to cool completely.

5. In a food processor or a large bowl, combine the cheesecake filling ingredients and mix on low speed or gently until smooth. (Don't whip—you don't want to add air.) Let the mixture set for 10 minutes to settle and allow any air bubbles to pop.

6. Pour the cheesecake mixture into the pan and use a rubber spatula to spread it evenly over the crust. Bake for 35 to 45 minutes, until the center just starts to firm up and the sides pull away. Let the cheesecake cool on the countertop for 1 hour, or until slightly above room temperature, then refrigerate until chilled through.

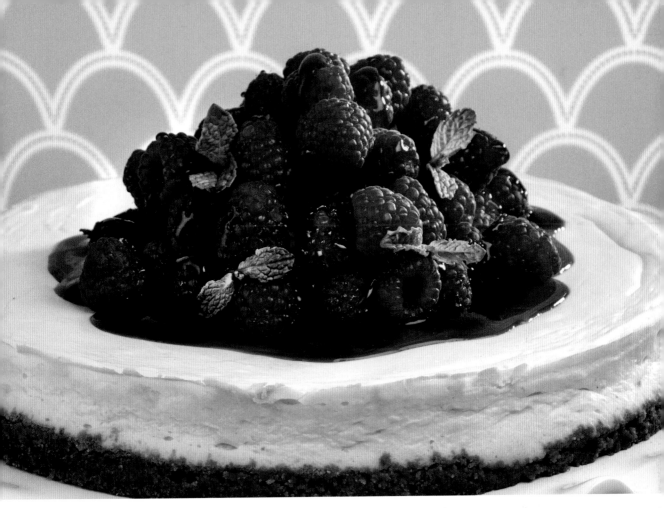

7. Meanwhile, combine the raspberry sauce ingredients in a blender and blend until all the berries are broken down into a liquid. Filter the sauce through a fine-mesh sieve into a small bowl to remove the seeds, then set it aside in the fridge until you're ready to serve the cheesecake.

8. When the cake is thoroughly chilled, gently release and remove the sides of the springform pan and place the cheesecake on a cake stand. Drizzle and splatter the top with the raspberry sauce, or pour it all on and smooth over the top (if you're traveling with this, hold off on the sauce until you reach your destination). Use a large, sharp knife to cut the cheesecake into sixteen servings.

If you prefer strawberry or blueberry sauce, simply swap the raspberries for your favorite berry. You can even make all three options and put them in gravy boats next to your cheesecake. This will give your guests options—and while you're at it, put out bowls of extra berries, too.

To make smaller amounts of these three different toppings, cut the berries down to ½ cup, the sugar to 1 tablespoon, and the lemon juice to ¼ teaspoon (adding more as needed to thin the sauces).

Tiramisu

Makes 6 servings
Serving size: 1 slice
Per serving: calories 82; fat 0.5 g; fiber 0 g; protein 7 g; carbohydrates 13 g

I think tiramisu is the ultimate naughty dessert, made even more delicious by eating it in bed with your better half. (Hey, I said naughty, didn't I?) My husband and I often take our restaurant tiramisu home in a doggie bag for just this reason. My aunt has even stopped asking if I want my serving after Christmas dinner or packed up for "later"—she knows me too well!

But this romantic dessert typically contains more than 600 calories per serving. Even if you split it, it's hard to enjoy without guilt. So I created this yummy low-calorie tiramisu with Greek yogurt and significantly lowered the amount of sugar, cutting hundreds of calories without sacrificing flavor. Trust me, I have no issue eating the full-fat version of this delicious dessert on special occasions, but I've come to prefer my light, fluffy, skinny version.

12 ladyfinger cookies
1 cup strong brewed coffee or espresso, cold
1½ cups 0% Greek yogurt
2½ tablespoons powdered sugar
2 teaspoons unsweetened cocoa powder

1. In a glass pie pan, arrange a single layer of 6 ladyfinger cookies: 3 on one half and 3 on the other half (don't worry if there are gaps). Pour ½ cup cold coffee over the cookies, and set it aside to soak in while you make the filling.

2. In a small bowl, combine the yogurt and powdered sugar (the powdered sugar thickens it, so don't use fake sugar or the consistency will be all off). When the cookies have soaked up the coffee, spoon half the yogurt mixture over the cookies and spread it out evenly. Sift 1 teaspoon cocoa powder over the yogurt.

3. Lay the last 6 cookies on top, this time 4 across the middle and 1 on the top and 1 on the bottom. Drizzle over the remaining coffee, and let sit until the coffee has soaked in. Spread the remaining yogurt on top and sift the remaining cocoa powder over the yogurt.

4. Refrigerate for 30 minutes to 1 hour before serving. Slice it like a pie, scoop out two portions, light some candles, and put on some romantic tunes. Store in the fridge, covered, for up to 2 days.

NOTE: I made this recipe without alcohol so the entire family can enjoy it, but you can spike individual slices for the adults: put ½ teaspoon dark rum or amaretto on a plate and top with a slice of tiramisu. Within seconds the bottom cookie layer will soak up the alcohol and give a boozy kick, with only 5 or 6 more calories per slice.

To ensure your kids aren't wired on coffee into all hours of the night, use strongly brewed decaf.

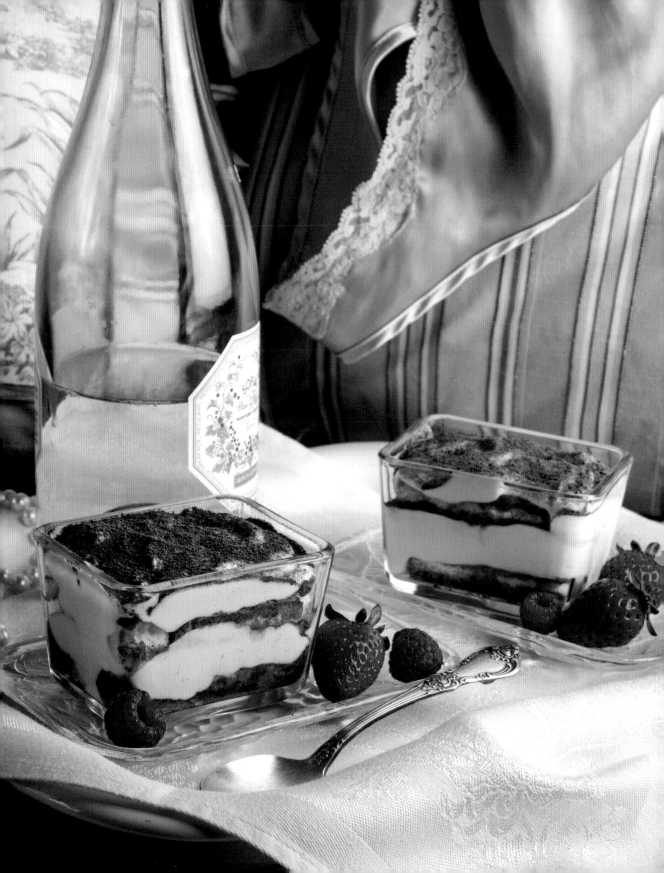

Strawberry Almond Oatmeal Crumble

Makes 6 servings
Serving size: about ⅔ cup
Per serving: calories 199; fat 3.5 g; fiber 9 g; protein 10 g; carbohydrates 55 g

I gave the average crumble recipe a makeover by adding ingredients that naturally help you lose weight. Strawberries, almonds, and oatmeal all naturally boost the metabolism, making this a recipe that works for you. The combination is great for backyard barbecues and has become a Fourth of July favorite at my house.

Filling

5 cups strawberries, quartered
1½ tablespoons granulated sugar
½ teaspoon pure almond extract
1 teaspoon pure vanilla extract

Crumble

1 cup old-fashioned rolled oats
3 tablespoons almond flour (if you don't
   have almond flour use all-purpose flour)
3 tablespoons slivered almonds
1 tablespoon granulated sugar
2 tablespoons light brown sugar
3 tablespoons Homemade Applesauce
   (page 112)
2 tablespoons unsalted butter, cold, cut into
   small pieces

1. Preheat the oven to 350°F.

2. Make the filling: In a large bowl, combine all the filling ingredients. Stir gently to combine and tumble the mixture into a 9 x 9-inch casserole dish.

3. Make the crumble: Wipe out the bowl and add the oats, almond flour, slivered almonds, and sugars. Mix to combine, then add the applesauce and butter. Mix with your fingers until the butter is in chunks the size of small peas and the mixture sticks together when you squeeze it between your fingers.

4. Crumble the topping over the filling and bake for 45 minutes, or until the topping is golden brown and the berries are bubbling. Set aside to cool for 25 minutes before serving to let the filling firm up.

Replace half the strawberries with blueberries, peach slices, or cranberries (great for holidays), or use a bag of frozen berry medley to keep it simple.

NOTE: I removed more than ½ cup granulated sugar from the original recipe, but if you like you can remove all the sugar from the topping and lightly sprinkle 1 teaspoon (just 16 calories!) over the top. Whatever you do, don't use artificial sweeteners; they'll turn this into a soupy mess. Use the real stuff.

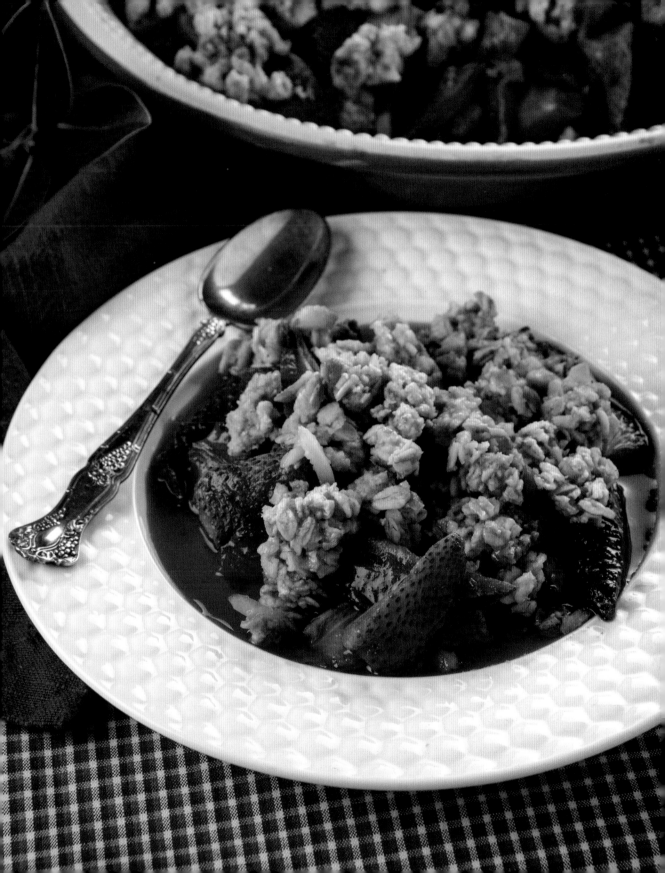

Peach Sunrise Cobbler

Makes 8 servings
Serving size: 1 slice
Per serving: calories 143; fat 10 g; fiber 2 g; protein 2 g; carbohydrates 18 g

I just adore this recipe, and I strongly advise you to bake it in a glass pie plate to fully enjoy its beauty. As the beautiful golden peaches cook, the almost fuchsia-colored raspberries bleed and create a stunning sunrise effect. You don't want to miss the view!

Unless you have a peach orchard in your backyard, go for frozen here and save yourself an hour of slicing and peeling. I took out more than ½ cup sugar from this recipe and cut the butter by more than half by incorporating applesauce.

Filling
3 cups frozen peach slices
½ cup fresh or frozen raspberries
1½ tablespoons granulated sugar
1 teaspoon pure vanilla extract

Crumble
1 cup old-fashioned rolled oats
3 tablespoons all-purpose flour
1 tablespoon granulated sugar
1 tablespoon light brown sugar
3 tablespoons Homemade Applesauce
   (page 112)
2 tablespoons unsalted butter, cold, cut into
   small pieces

1. Preheat the oven to 350°F.

2. Make the filling: In a large bowl, combine all the filling ingredients. Stir gently to combine and tumble the mixture into a pie pan.

3. Make the crumble: Wipe out the bowl and add the oats, flour, and sugars. Mix to combine, then add the applesauce and butter. Mix with your fingers until the butter is in chunks the size of small peas and the mixture sticks together when you squeeze it between your fingers.

4. Crumble the topping over the peaches and bake for 40 minutes, or until the topping is golden brown and the filling is bubbling. Set aside to cool for 25 minutes before serving to let the filling firm up.

NOTE: Don't use artificial sweeteners; they'll turn the dish into a soupy mess.

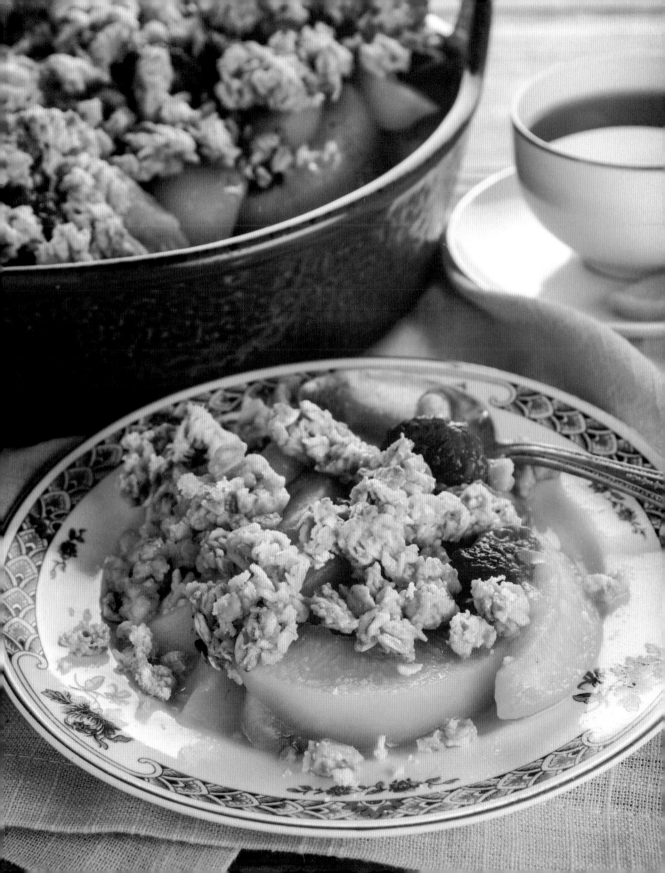

Strawberry Shortcake Cupcakes

Makes 24 cupcakes
Serving size: 1 cupcake
Per serving: calories 130; fat 8 g; fiber 1 g; protein 3 g; carbohydrates 15 g

I was walking through the produce section of my local grocery store and came across the familiar strawberry display that comes with spring. Foamy, preservative-filled "cakes" and sugary chocolate and caramel tubs lined the sides of the display. Of course my daughter wanted all of it, but strawberries were the only thing in this display that belonged in the produce section.

I decided this would be the perfect opportunity for a baking lesson with my little girl. We got two 1-pound cartons of strawberries (one to bake with and one to nibble on while we worked) and grabbed some organic whipping cream. Instead of spending fifteen or twenty dollars on the display items, I spent eight dollars and got three times the strawberries.

If you've never made your own sweetened whipped cream, prepare yourself for the best thing ever! All you need is two ingredients: a whisk and a smile.

Cupcakes
Olive oil spray
1½ cups self-rising flour
¼ teaspoon kosher salt
1 teaspoon baking soda
¾ cup 0% Greek yogurt
1½ cups strawberries, sliced
½ cup unsweetened almond milk
3 large eggs
½ cup granulated sugar

Topping
2 cups heavy cream
3 tablespoons powdered sugar
18 fresh strawberries, hulled and quartered

1. Preheat the oven to 350°F. Lightly spray two 12-cup cupcake pans with olive oil.

2. Make the cupcakes: In a medium bowl, combine the flour, salt, and baking soda. Mix and set aside.

3. In a blender or food processor, combine the yogurt, strawberries, and almond milk. Blend until smooth.

4. In the bowl of a stand mixer fitted with the paddle attachment or in a large bowl, whisk the eggs and granulated sugar until pale and fluffy, about 5 minutes. Mix in half the flour mixture until just incorporated, then the strawberry mixture until just incorporated, then the remaining flour mixture until all the ingredients are incorporated. Don't overmix or the cupcakes will be tough.

5. Using an ice cream scoop, fill the cupcake molds three-quarters full of batter. (If there are any empty wells in the pans, add a little water to them so they don't burn.) Bake for 18 to 25 minutes, or until a toothpick inserted into the center of a cupcake comes out clean. Set the cupcakes aside to cool completely before topping them.

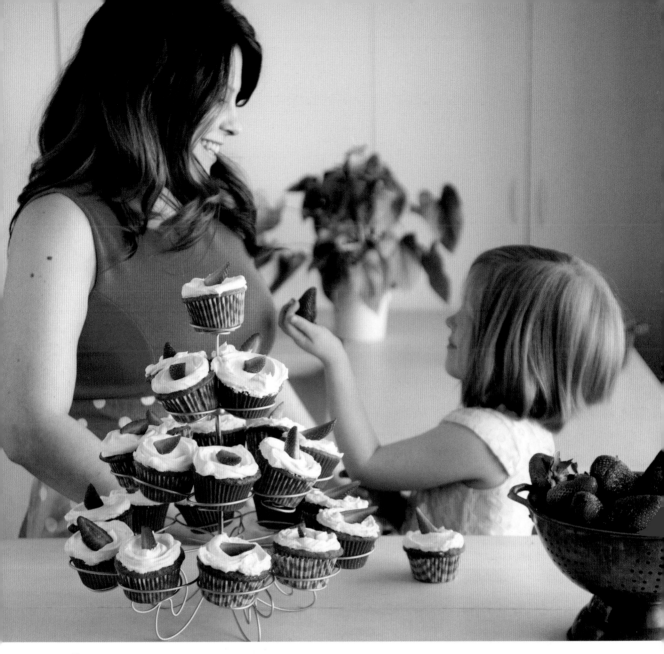

6. Make the topping: In a large bowl or the bowl of the stand mixer fitted with the whisk attachment, whisk the heavy cream and powdered sugar until firm peaks form, 3 to 5 minutes.

7. If you're serving the cupcakes immediately, top each with 2 strawberry quarters and 2 tablespoons of the whipped cream. Dot the whipped cream with a single strawberry quarter. Keep the rest of the cupcakes, cut strawberries, and whipped cream in the fridge until you're ready to serve them. The whipped cream will keep separately but not on the cupcakes.

Champagne Cupcakes with Orange and Raspberry Buttercream Frosting

Makes 24 cupcakes
Serving size: 1 cupcake
Per serving: calories 154; fat 3 g; fiber 0.5 g; protein 1 g; carbohydrates 28 g

These champagne cupcakes aren't for your kid's birthday party; they pack an elegant punch as a dessert at cocktail or dinner parties. Make mini-cupcakes for brunch buffets, or toast the New Year with a cupcake instead of a glass of bubbly.

The cake part of these cupcakes is beautifully brut and not very sweet. The sweet orange frosting gives a mimosa effect and the tart raspberry frosting gives you a Chambord cupcake. You get the best of both worlds—a glass of bubbly in the form of a cupcake!

Cupcakes
Butter wrapper or olive oil spray
2 cups all-purpose flour
¾ cup granulated sugar
¼ teaspoon baking powder
½ teaspoon baking soda
2 cups champagne, prosecco, or sparkling white wine
½ cup Homemade Applesauce (page 112)
¼ cup unsweetened almond milk

Raspberry Frosting
4 tablespoons (½ stick) unsalted butter, at room temperature
1½ cups powdered sugar
1 tablespoon raspberry jam

Orange Frosting
4 tablespoons (½ stick) unsalted butter, at room temperature
1½ cups powdered sugar
1 tablespoon orange juice concentrate

Fresh raspberries (optional)
Orange slices (optional)

1. Preheat the oven to 350°F. Grease two 12-cup muffin tins with the inside of a butter wrapper, or if you're using paper liners, spray them with olive oil spray.

2. Make the cupcakes: In a large bowl, combine the flour, sugar, baking powder, and baking soda. Slowly pour in the champagne so it doesn't bubble over, then add the applesauce and gently mix together with a spatula or spoon (not a mixer). When the mixture is mostly combined, add the almond milk and mix until there are no lumps. Don't overmix, as it will make tough cupcakes.

3. Pour the batter into the tins and bake for 14 to 18 minutes, or until the cupcakes are firm to the touch and a toothpick inserted into the center of a cupcake comes out clean. Let the cupcakes cool in the pans for 15 minutes, then refrigerate for at least 20 minutes to cool completely while you make the frosting.

4. Make the raspberry frosting: In the bowl of a stand mixer fitted with the whisk attachment or in a large bowl with a whisk, whisk the butter, sugar, raspberry jam, and 1 teaspoon warm water until the frosting starts to ball up on the whisk. If necessary, add warm water 1 teaspoon at a time until you reach the desired consistency; you want it thick enough not to run or drip.

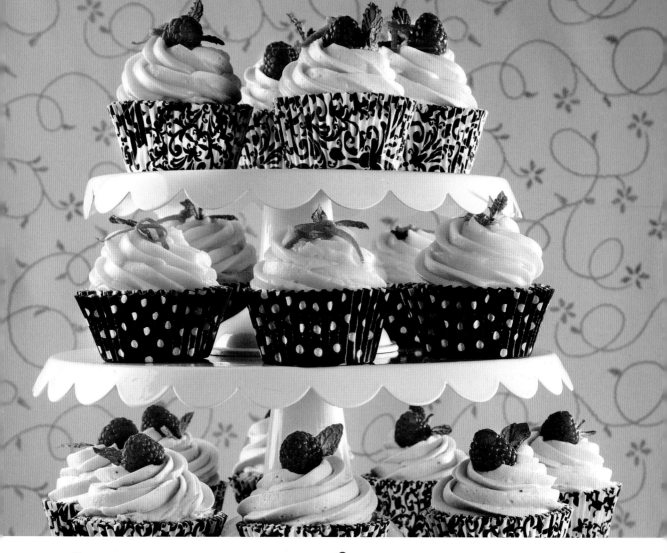

5. Make the orange frosting: In the bowl of a stand mixer fitted with the whisk attachment or in a large bowl with a whisk, whisk the butter, sugar, orange juice concentrate, and 1 teaspoon warm water until the frosting starts to ball up on the whisk. If needed, add 1 teaspoon warm water at a time until you reach the right consistency; you want it thick enough not to run or drip.

6. With a decorating bag or a spoon, top 12 of the cupcakes with the raspberry frosting and 12 with the orange frosting. Let the cupcakes sit for a couple of minutes, then garnish them with fresh raspberries or orange slices, if desired. Refrigerate for 30 minutes to set the frosting. Store covered in the fridge for up to 3 days.

NOTE: This recipe will make 48 mini cupcakes . . . and that's a lot! If you don't need 48 mini cupcakes, cut the recipe in half and you'll have 24 mini cupcakes. Bake for 8 to 10 minutes—these babies don't need as much time as the big mamas do.

Apple Pie Squares

Makes 12 servings
Serving size: 1 square
Per serving: calories 93; fat 4 g; fiber 1 g; protein 0 g; carbohydrates 15 g

---

I adore apple pie, but the average slice has around 450 calories. That's an entire meal for me, so I gave this old favorite a skinny makeover. I shaved hundreds of calories plus extra fat and sugar from this recipe with just a few Simple Swaps. First, my crust is so easy and delicious that you'll never buy premade again. I cut the calories, sugar, and fat with the help of applesauce, which adds sweetness and replaces some of the butter. Second, I chose sweet apples over tart and added lots of cinnamon, nutmeg, and ginger to pack in flavor. By using sweet apples like Fuji, Gala, or Honeycrisp, you won't need as much sugar to sweeten this dish. The result is an apple pie square that's so low in calories that you can enjoy it with a scoop of organic vanilla ice cream or a slice of cheddar cheese without blowing your daily calories.

Crust
½ cup Homemade Applesauce (page 112)
4 tablespoons (½ stick) unsalted butter,
    at room temperature
¼ cup granulated sugar
1 teaspoon pure vanilla extract
Kosher salt
1½ cups all-purpose flour

Filling
5 apples, peeled, cored, and thinly sliced
2 tablespoons dark brown sugar
1 teaspoon ground cinnamon
¼ teaspoon ground ginger
¼ teaspoon ground nutmeg
    (freshly grated, if you have it)

1. Preheat the oven to 350°F. Line a 9 x 9-inch casserole dish with parchment paper.

2. Make the crust: In a large bowl or the bowl of a stand mixer fitted with the paddle attachment, combine the applesauce, butter, and granulated sugar and whisk until creamy and fluffy. Add the vanilla, a pinch of salt, and the flour and mix until combined and crumbly.

3. Pour half the crust mixture into the prepared dish and press it into a thin layer over the bottom and up the sides of the casserole dish with a rubber spatula or wet hands.

4. Make the filling: In a large bowl, combine the filling ingredients and toss until the apple slices are well coated.

5. Tumble the filling into the crust and spread it out in an even layer. Use your fingers to crumble the remaining crust over the apples, and fold any excess dough on the sides over the top.

6. Bake for 30 to 35 minutes, until the topping is browned and crunchy. Set aside to cool for 30 minutes to let the bottom of the crust continue cooking. Slice into twelve squares and serve, or refrigerate for later and slice when you're ready to serve.

Dark Chocolate–Covered Fruit

Makes 36 servings
Serving size: 1 piece of chocolate-covered fruit
Per serving with fresh fruit: calories 22; fat 1 g; fiber 0.5 g;
protein 0.5 g; carbohydrates 3.5 g
Per serving with dried fruit: calories 35; fat 1 g; fiber 1 g, protein 0.5 g; carbohydrates 6 g

---

When I originally set out to write a skinny fondue recipe, I realized that between the chocolate and the heavy cream, cutting the calories was next to impossible, so I decided to create the next best thing: chocolate-covered fruit. Plus, you can make these ahead of time and store them in your freezer—you can't do that with a pot of hot, bubbling chocolate!

½ cup dark chocolate chips
1 teaspoon olive oil

Fresh Fruit
1 apple, cored and cut into 12 slices
1 banana, cut into 12 slices
12 strawberries

Dried Fruit
6 dried peaches, halved
3 dried pineapple rings, quartered
12 dried banana chips

1. Clear a space in the freezer. Cover a baking sheet with waxed paper and place the chosen fruit on the prepared sheet.

2. In a double boiler or a heatproof bowl over (but not touching) a pan one-third full of boiling water, melt the chocolate. Use a rubber spatula to gently mix so that the chocolate doesn't burn. When the chocolate is fully melted, turn off the heat and mix in the oil (be sure to use an oven mitt while handling the bowl).

3. Use a spoon to drizzle the chocolate over the fruit, starting slow with a little on each slice and adding more as you go.

4. Freeze for at least 10 to 20 minutes before serving.

Pineapple Mango Ginger Sorbet

Makes 7 servings
Serving size: ⅓ cup
Per serving: calories 60; fat 0 g; fiber 1 g; protein 0 g; carbohydrates 15 g

This sorbet is simply amazing. The pineapple makes it super sweet without adding extra sugar, the mango adds smoothness, and the ginger ale gives a kick of muted spice, making it a nicely complex dessert. If ginger ale is too spicy for your kids, just use all-natural lemon-lime soda or sparkling water.

What makes this dessert extra special is that all three ingredients naturally boost your metabolism! This fat-burning dessert is a great way to curb your sweet tooth while getting a boost of vitamin C—and it's great for colds, too! Have a sore throat? Try some cool sorbet. With all the nutrients in this dessert, you can almost call it a cold buster!

1 cup frozen pineapple chunks
1 cup frozen mango chunks
1 bottle all-natural ginger ale or
    ginger beer

1. Blend all the ingredients in a blender or food processor until smooth.

2. Pour the mixture into a 9 x 9-inch glass dish and freeze for 1 hour. Scrape the frozen mixture thoroughly with a fork. Repeat twice: freeze for 2 more hours, scraping twice.

3. Transfer the sorbet to a plastic container and store it in your freezer for up to 1 month.

Peach Mint Sorbet: Use 2 cups frozen peaches in place of the pineapple and mango, and a can of organic lemon-lime soda (Hansen's is good) in place of the ginger ale, and add 5 mint leaves.

Spiked Sorbet: Swap in sparkling wine for the ginger ale.

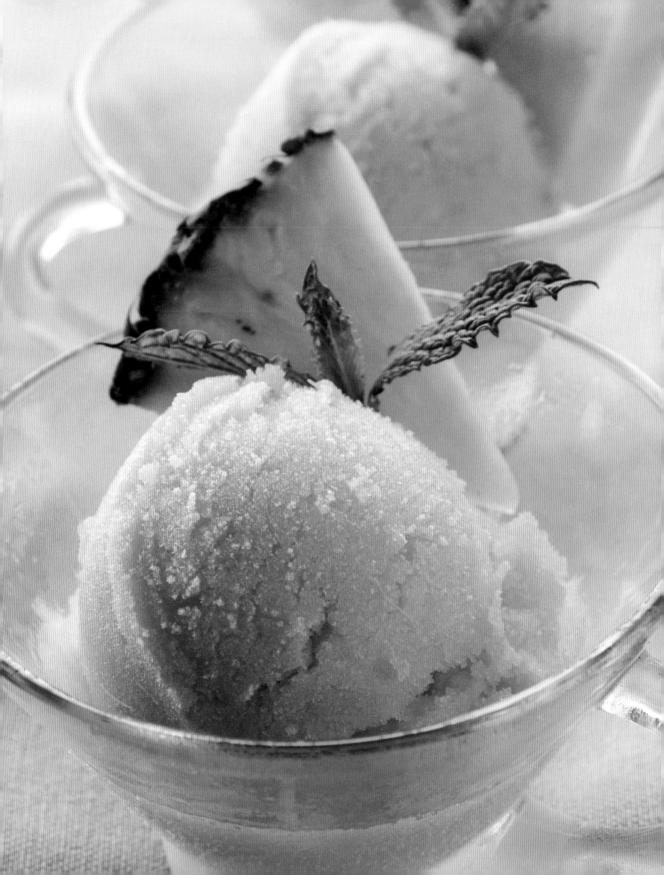

Orange Cream Ice Pops

Makes 4 ice pops
Serving size: 1 ice pop
Per serving: calories 61; fat 0 g; fiber 0 g; protein 5 g; carbohydrates 8 g

---

I love those unhealthy orange cream frozen treats you find in the freezer section, but I won't buy them anymore. All the artificial colors, preservatives, and chemical thickeners actually harm your weight-loss results, especially the ones labeled sugar-free! Now these creamy, tangy ice pops are full of good-for-you ingredients, like metabolism-boosting Greek yogurt and vitamin C–packed oranges, and will actually help your weight loss rather than impede it.

There are only 2 tablespoons powdered sugar in four pops, but if you really don't want to use real sugar, try honey or just skip it altogether. Whatever you do, avoid the nasty fake stuff!

¾ cup 0% Greek yogurt
2 tablespoons frozen orange juice concentrate
2 tablespoons powdered sugar
1½ teaspoons pure vanilla extract
1 orange

1. In a blender, puree the yogurt, orange juice concentrate, sugar, and vanilla until smooth.

2. Peel the orange (discard the peel and seeds) and drop the segments into the blender, letting the juices spill in, too, as you work. Pulse until the fruit is in small chunks.

3. Pour the mixture into ice pop molds and freeze until solid, about 6 to 8 hours.

4. Pull the ice pops out of the freezer 5 to 10 minutes before serving so that they unmold easily.

Tangerines and Cream: Substitute 2 tangerines for the orange.

Berries and Cream: Swap in 10 strawberries and 1 banana for the orange juice concentrate and orange. Fold ½ cup chopped berries into the blender mixture before pouring it into the molds.

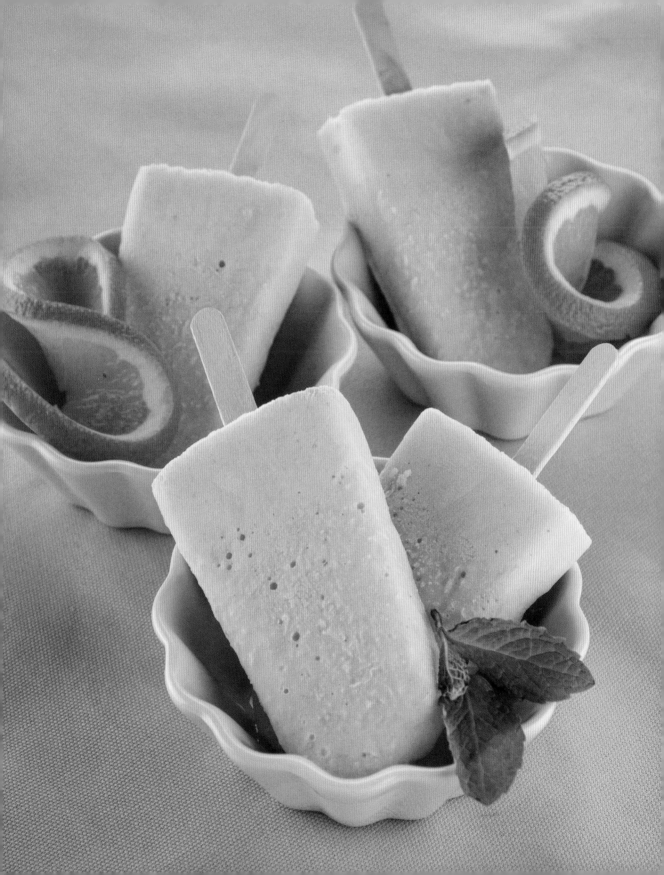

Loaded Chocolate-Covered Bananas

Makes 4 banana pops
Serving size: 1 banana pop
Per serving without toppings: calories 125; fat 5 g;
fiber 2.5 g; protein 1.5 g; carbohydrates 22 g
Per serving with Almond Roca Topping: calories 169; fat 9 g;
fiber 3 g; protein 2.5 g; carbohydrates 24 g

When I was a kid, it didn't get any better than frozen chocolate-covered bananas on a hot day! I use dark chocolate instead of milk chocolate to cut calories, fat, and sugar and opt for all-natural chewy and crunchy toppings with health benefits.

Banana Pops

¼ cup dark chocolate or semisweet chocolate chips
1 teaspoon olive oil
4 whole mini bananas or 2 large bananas, halved

Almond Roca Topping

1 tablespoon unsweetened coconut flakes, toasted
1 tablespoon chopped toasted almonds

1. Clear a space in the freezer. Cover a baking sheet with waxed paper.

2. In a double boiler or a heatproof bowl over (but not touching) a pan one-third full of boiling water, melt the chocolate. Use a rubber spatula to gently mix so that the chocolate doesn't burn. When the chocolate is fully melted, turn off the heat and mix in the oil (be sure to use an oven mitt while handling the bowl).

3. Let's make the bananas! Add the topping ingredients to a pie plate (I combine them all together in one plate, but if you have a picky eater who doesn't like one ingredient, you can move that one ingredient to another pie plate and dip it separately). Peel the bananas and skewer them with ice pop sticks, chopsticks, or wooden skewers with the sharp ends cut off. Dip a banana into the chocolate, using a rubber spatula to help cover it with chocolate, and hold it for a second over the bowl to let the excess drip back in. Dunk the banana into the toppings and place it on the prepared cookie sheet. Repeat with the rest of the bananas.

4. Drizzle any leftover melted chocolate over the prepared bananas.

5. Freeze the bananas on the tray for 4 hours, or until the bananas are frozen and the chocolate is set. Move any extras to a freezer bag and store for up to 1 month in your freezer.

Hawaiian: Swap the almonds for 1 tablespoon chopped dried pineapple and 1 tablespoon chopped macadamia nuts.

Cherry Almond: Skip the Almond Roca Topping and use 1 tablespoon chopped dried cherries and 1 tablespoon toasted slivered almonds.

PB&J: Instead of the Almond Roca Topping, use 1 tablespoon chopped dried strawberries and 1 tablespoon chopped lightly salted peanuts.

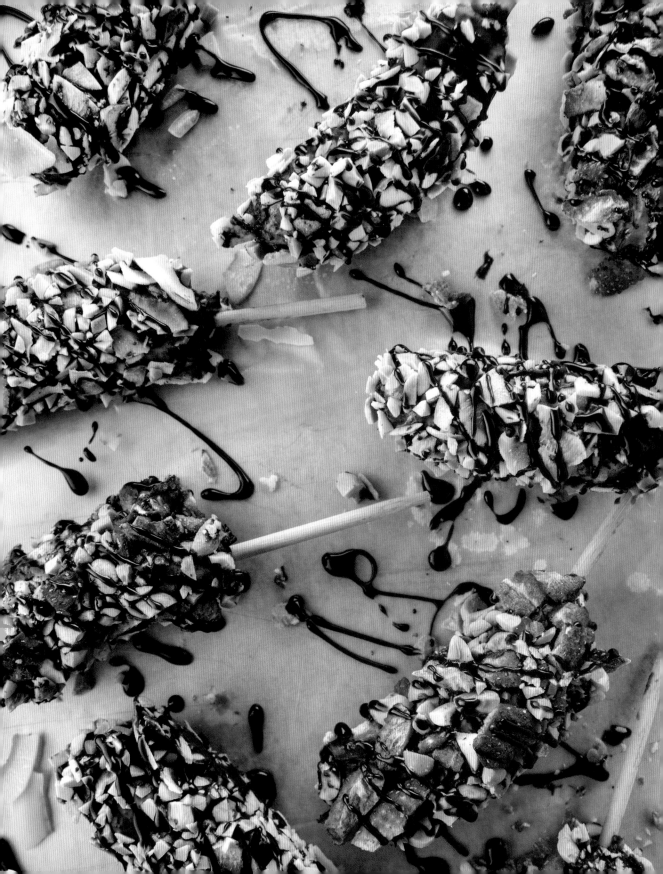

Chapter 14

Skinny Drinks

You hear it all the time: *Don't drink your calories.* People get frustrated when they're dieting and the pounds aren't coming off, but often they don't realize that their beloved diet soda is causing weight gain and their favorite sugary juice is adding empty calories.

The purpose of this chapter is to wean you off diet-busting choices and help you fall in love with drinks that love you back. You'll find drinks to help you get to a gallon of water a day, coffee drinks to give you a jolt of energy in the A.M., and cocktails for a homemade happy hour.

My favorite Smart Swaps for this chapter:

Almond milk is great in coffee drinks; even the unsweetened variety adds
creaminess and sweetness!

Greek yogurt adds creaminess and thickens drinks without loads of calories.

Grand Marnier and orange liqueur add sweetness and a blast of flavor. A
little goes a long way, so use sparingly.

Homemade Blueberry Orange Soda

Makes 8 servings
Serving size: ½ liter
Per serving: calories 3.5; fat 0 g; fiber 0 g; protein 0 g; carbohydrates 1 g
(nutrition based on infused water only, not consuming the fruit)

Do you have a soda addiction? It's okay to admit it—I did, too. The week I gave up diet soda I lost ten pounds without even trying, and I found that it wasn't the sweetness I craved in diet soda but the bubbles.

Whenever I crave soda now, I throw some frozen blueberries in sparkling water, and within a few seconds, my craving is met—all while I'm meeting my daily water goal. Frozen blueberries pop and bleed the second you add them to sparkling water, giving it a stunning purple hue. I add orange slices for extra vitamin C and a metabolism boost, but any citrus will work well here—just use what you have on hand.

4 liters sparkling water
2 oranges, cut into thin slices
2 cups frozen blueberries
½ cup fresh mint leaves (optional)

1. If serving immediately, pour the sparkling water into one large pitcher or two small pitchers. If serving later, leave the water in the bottles and pour some out to make room for the fruit. (I drink it from a wineglass while I'm making the recipe.)

2. Add the orange slices and blueberries to the bubbly water. If using small pitchers or bottles, divide the fruit among the containers. If the bottle opening is small, roll the orange slices up and slide them into the opening. Do the same with the mint leaves, squeezing them as you drop them into the water. This will help release the oils and add more flavor.

3. Serve immediately or close and tighten the lids. Infuse for 2 hours for maximum flavor.

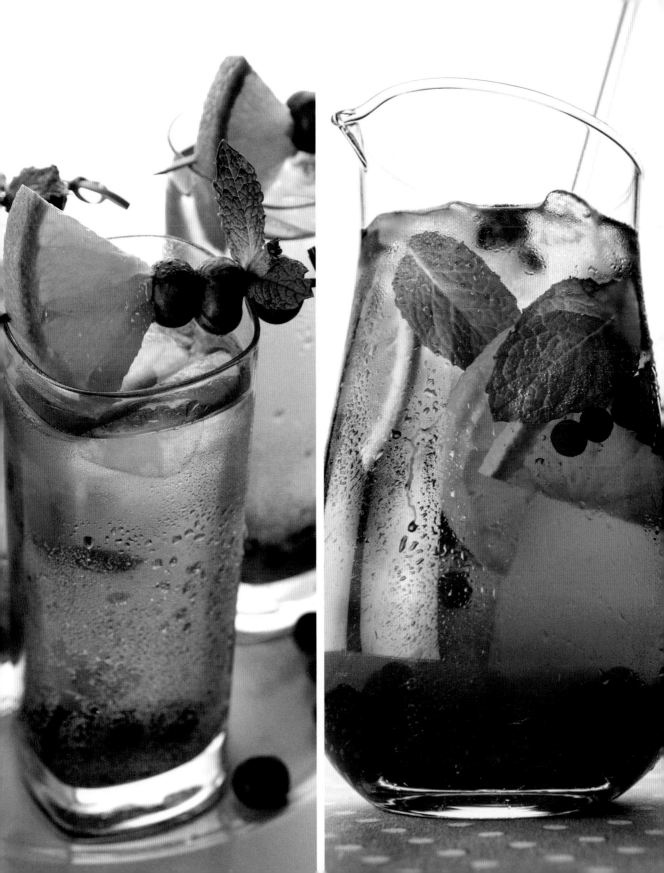

Skin-Firming Citrus Boost Water

Makes 1 gallon (8 cups)
Serving size: 2 cups
Per serving: calories 5; fat 0 g; fiber 0 g; protein 0 g; carbohydrates 1 g
(nutrition based on infused water only, not consuming the fruit)

Bored of plain flat water? Try adding some fruit! This water is one of my personal favorites. I like to make it at night before I go to bed. I awake to a delicious, full-flavored drink with abundant health and beauty benefits. Mangoes and citrus boost your metabolism, and they're also known to help naturally smooth and tighten skin. Drink as much as you like—remember, you're trying to drink a gallon of water a day, and this will make your goal deliciously possible to meet.

2 mangoes
2 oranges, cut into slices
1 lemon, cut into slices
1 lime, cut into slices
4 cups ice

1. Peel and cut the mangoes into large chunks, reserving the pits. Divide the mango chunks between two large pitchers. Squeeze the excess juice off the pits and drop them in as well. Add the citrus slices and top with the ice, which will hold down the fruit. Pour in 1 gallon water.

2. Let the water infuse for at least 2 hours before serving or store overnight in your fridge. If you like your water at room temperature, let it infuse on the countertop, but be sure to add the ice to hold down the fruit, or use a fruit infusion pitcher, which will hold all the fruit down for you without the ice.

NOTE: Check out my favorite fruit infusion water pitchers on my website, loseweightbyeating.com.

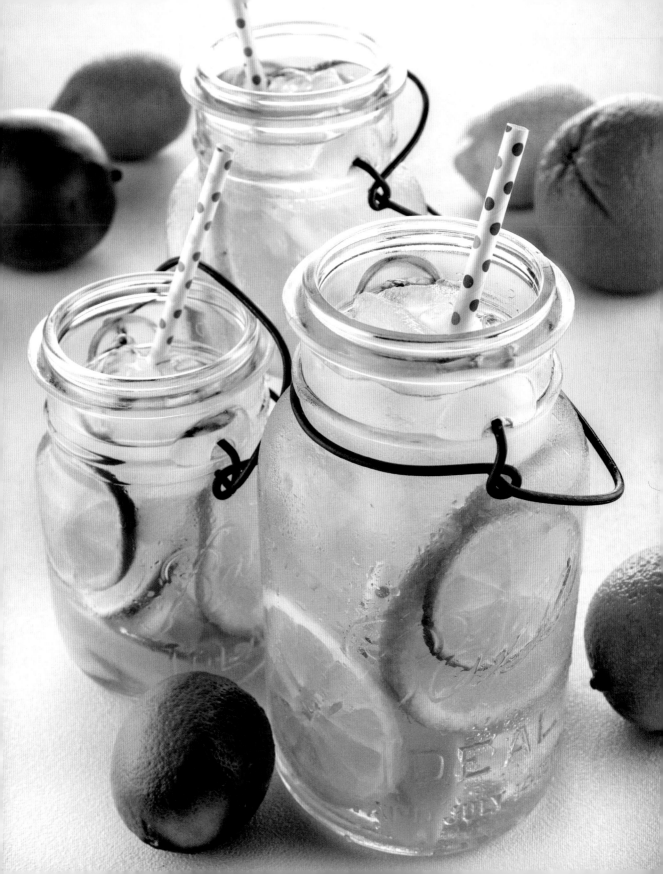

Berry Medley Mint Water

Makes 1 serving
Serving size: one (16-ounce) glass
Per serving: calories 2; fat 0 g; fiber 0 g; protein 0 g; carbohydrates 0 g
(nutrition based on infused water only, not consuming the fruit)

Here's a five-minute recipe you can enjoy right away as a single glass or let infuse overnight in a larger quantity (see Note). The longer the fruit and mint infuse, the more flavorful the drink. You can also double down on flavor— infuse the water and add a handful of frozen berries in lieu of ice and a couple of fresh mint leaves to your glass.

This thirst quencher is good for all ages— pregnant and nursing moms, too! So drink up!

⅛ cup frozen mixed berries
2 fresh mint leaves

1. Add the berries to a glass. Squeeze the mint a little to release the oils and drop it into the glass. Top with 2 cups water and enjoy.

NOTE: To make a larger amount, use 2 cups frozen mixed berries, ½ cup fresh mint leaves, 4 cups ice, and 1 gallon water. Add the berries and mint to a gallon pitcher (or divide between two smaller pitchers). Top with ice to hold down the fruit and finish by adding the water. Let the water infuse for at least 2 hours before serving or overnight in your fridge. If you like your water at room temperature, let it infuse on the countertop, but be sure to add the ice to hold down the fruit, or use a fruit infusion pitcher. This recipe makes 8 servings.

Blueberry Mint Vodka Spritzers

Makes 6 liters, 25 servings
Serving size: one (8-ounce) glass
Per serving: calories 62; fat 0 g; fiber 0.5 g; protein 0 g; carbohydrates 10 g

These Blueberry Mint Vodka Spritzers can be made without vodka. They're a refreshing drink to sip by the pool on a hot afternoon or a great cocktail to serve at a backyard barbecue.

3 cups blueberries (frozen or fresh will work here)
½ cup honey
Juice of 7 lemons
8 fresh mint leaves
Juice of 1 orange
4 liters sparkling water or club soda, chilled
2 ounces (¼ cup) Grand Marnier (optional)
1 cup vodka, chilled (optional)

1. In a medium saucepan, combine the blueberries, honey, and ⅓ cup water over medium-high heat. Cook, stirring often, until all the blueberries pop, about 8 minutes.

2. Pour the blueberry syrup into a blender and add the lemon juice, mint, and orange juice. Blend until smooth. Refrigerate until chilled.

3. When you're ready to serve, combine the blueberry mixture, club soda, and Grand Marnier and vodka, if using, in a large punch bowl or two pitchers for easy pouring (you can make one with alcohol and one without). Mix and serve immediately so you don't lose your bubbles.

Blended Mocha Coffee

Makes 2 servings
Serving size: about 1½ cups
Per serving: calories 138; fat 3 g; fiber 2.5 g; protein 2.5 g; carbohydrates 26 g

I started making this as a way to use up my morning coffee. After a while I upped the ante and started freezing some of the leftover coffee into ice cubes for the next day's drink; you just throw them into a freezer bag and pull them out as needed. Coffee ice cubes are great in iced coffee and in an iced version of my Vanilla Latte (page 268).

Homemade Chocolate Syrup makes this a breeze!

1 cup strong black coffee, or 2 shots espresso, chilled
1 cup unsweetened almond milk
2 tablespoons 0% Greek yogurt
1 tablespoon semisweet chocolate chips
1 cup frozen coffee cubes or plain ice cubes
3 tablespoons Chocolate Syrup (see below)

1. Combine all the ingredients in a blender and blend until smooth, 1 to 2 minutes. Pour into two glasses and serve.

Chocolate Syrup

Makes 18 servings
Serving size: 1 tablespoon
Per serving: calories 42; fat 0 g; fiber 1 g; protein 0 g; carbohydrates 11 g

1½ cups sugar
1 cup unsweetened cocoa powder
⅛ teaspoon salt
1 teaspoon pure vanilla extract

1. In a medium saucepan, combine the 1½ cups water, the sugar, cocoa powder, and salt. Cook over medium heat, whisking continuously, until thickened, about 10 minutes. Whisk in the vanilla and remove from the heat. Store the syrup in a glass jar in the fridge for up to 1 month.

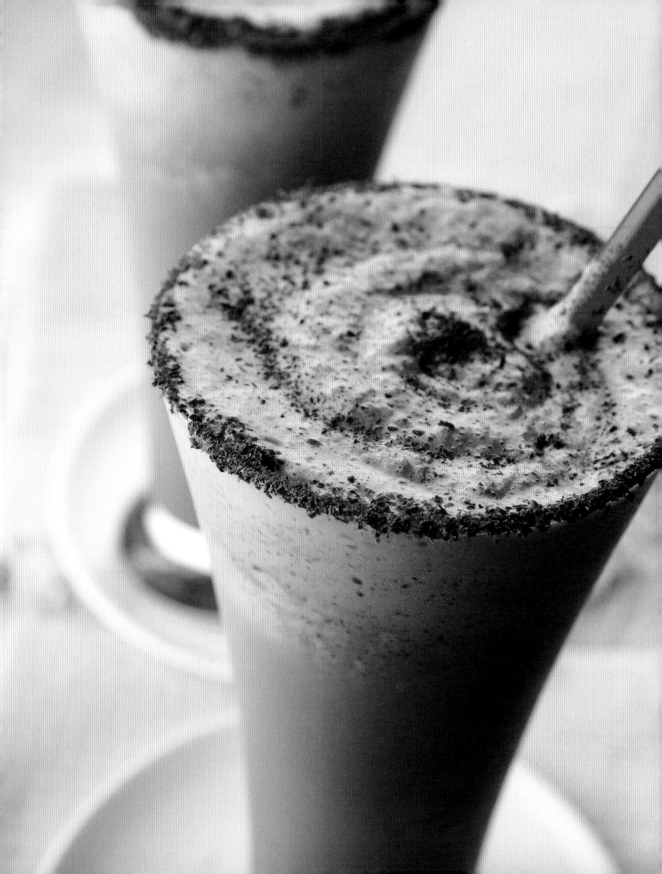

Vanilla Latte

Makes 2 lattes
Serving size: 1 latte
Per serving: calories 34; fat 1 g; fiber 0.5 g; protein 0.5 g; carbohydrates 4 g

An average coffeehouse vanilla latte is 250 calories, and the lower-calorie versions have more than 150 calories and are full of chemicals in place of sugar. Not to mention that these drinks can cost between three and five dollars each! These numbers cut so deeply into my daily calorie and money budgets that of course I had to invent my own version. All you need is a coffeemaker and a whisk, and you don't need to leave your PJs to make it.

1 cup unsweetened almond milk
½ teaspoon pure vanilla extract
1 cup strongly brewed coffee, hot

1. In a small saucepan, heat the almond milk over medium-low heat until warmed to taste. Whisk briskly and continuously until foamy, 1 to 2 minutes.

2. Remove from the heat and stir in the vanilla and coffee. Serve hot, or pour over ice for an iced vanilla latte.

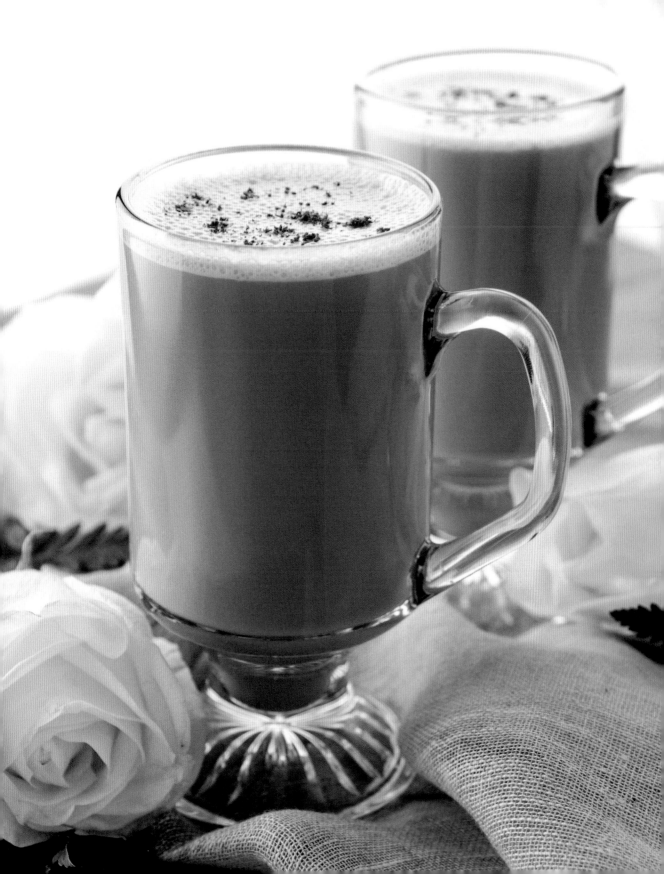

Watermelon Margaritas

Makes 4 margaritas
Serving size: 1 cup
Per serving: calories 116; fat 0 g; fiber 0.5 g; protein 1 g; carbohydrates 15 g

I spent one glorious summer vacation with my family on the beaches of Kitty Hawk, North Carolina, and made these Watermelon Margaritas on day two of our eight-day trip. As a reward, I was forced to make them every day after that; even my mother-in-law, who rarely drinks, couldn't stop asking for them. So whether you want to be the "favorite" relative or just need a delicious stress buster, get yourself a watermelon, a bottle of silver tequila, and your favorite orange liqueur and go to town.

Some tips for this recipe:

Be sure to get a seedless watermelon; you don't want to be seeding the thing for hours or, worse, picking black dots from your drink.

I prefer Grand Marnier, but any orange liqueur will work here; just get your personal favorite or what's on sale.

I highly recommend that you use silver tequila; the gold is far too pungent a flavor for this drink, and a milder flavor means you won't be tempted to add calories via sugar or agave.

An average watermelon (15 pounds), a standard bottle of tequila (750 mL), and a standard bottle of Grand Marnier (750 mL) will make about sixty margaritas, but the recipe below makes a four-margarita pitcher, to get you started. Freeze the rest of the watermelon in freezer bags (4 cups each) for instant margaritas any time.

Make this easy recipe even easier: halve the watermelon and use an ice cream scoop to scoop out the watermelon—you can even get the kids to help here. Just be sure to scoop small balls of watermelon, not huge ones, or they won't blend well.

4 cups watermelon cubes
¼ cup silver tequila
¼ cup Grand Marnier or other orange liqueur
½ lime, cut into wedges (optional)

1. Place the watermelon chunks in a large freezer-safe plastic container and freeze them completely, 3 to 5 hours.

2. Add the frozen watermelon, tequila, and orange liqueur to a blender and blend until smooth. Divide among four glasses and serve with lime wedges.

Pineapple Jalapeño Margaritas: Use 4 cups frozen pineapple chunks and 1 or 2 seeded jalapeños in place of the watermelon.

Strawberry Margaritas: Use 4 cups frozen strawberries, 1 teaspoon balsamic vinegar (for sweetness and to cut the acid in the strawberries), and 1 teaspoon powdered sugar in place of the watermelon.

Virgin Margaritas: Swap the tequila and orange liqueur with ½ cup organic lemon-lime soda.

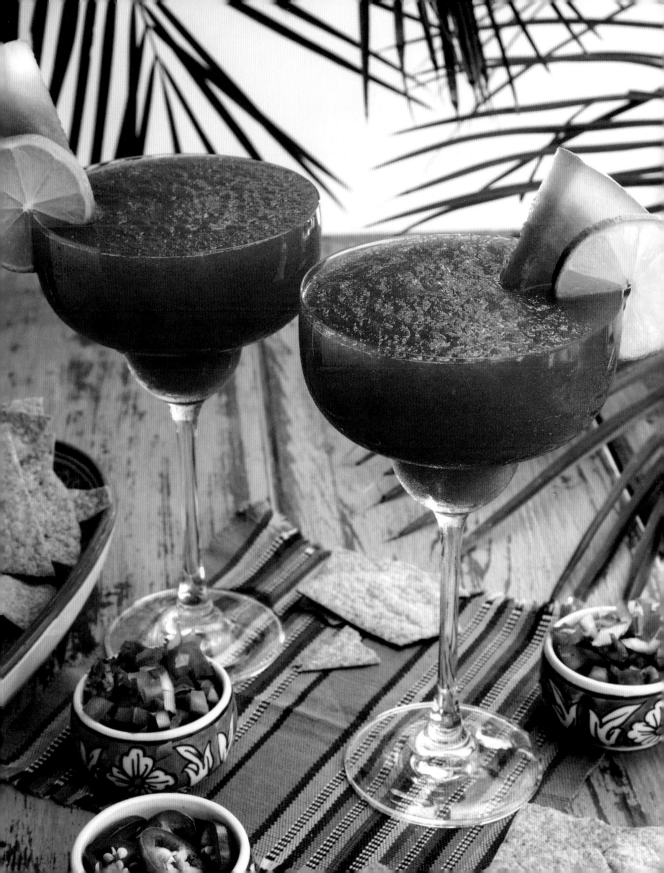

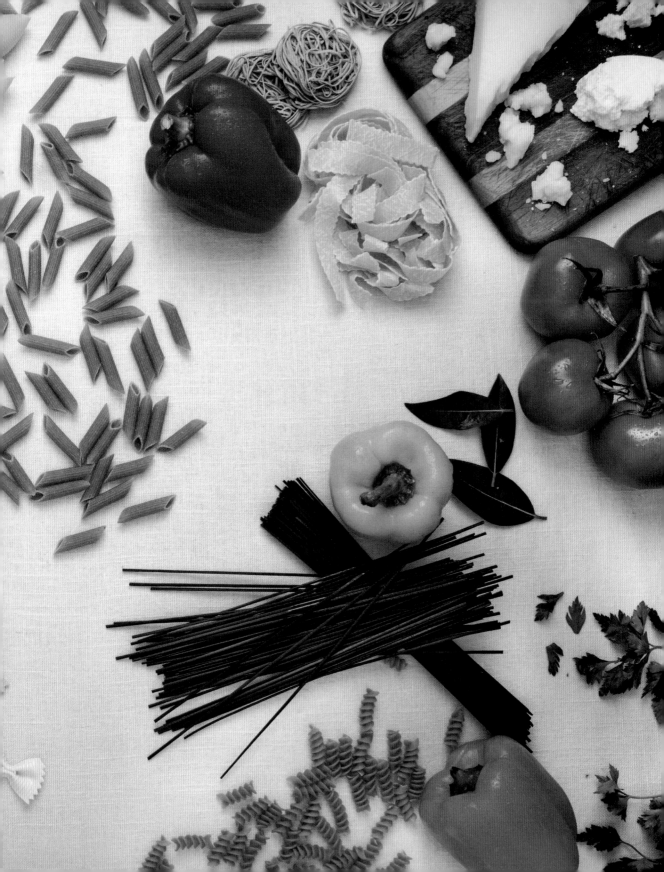

Meal Planners

So what does a week of food look like in the Lose Weight by Eating plan? I took the liberty of filling out six full-week meal planners for you. There's something for everyone, from new cooks to picky kids to vegetarians.

I recommend that you alternate the breakfast and lunch options to save money and time. For instance, if you're going to make granola, eat it two or three times this week for breakfast, not just once. I picked three options for breakfasts and lunches and alternated them so that you can use up the ingredients you already bought and stave off boredom. As for dinners, I picked seven for each menu, but you'll see that I use dinner leftovers as lunches—again it's all about saving you money and time.

Whenever you have leftovers, freeze them in individual portions for fast freezer dinners and lunches. This way, if you hit traffic on your way home from work and don't have time to cook, you can pull out a healthy premade meal and forget the stress. Those frozen dinners you get in your grocer's freezer section are full of preservatives, and the all-natural ones cost a fortune and never really fill you up. And freezing your leftovers will also keep you from nibbling on them at midnight!

METABOLISM-BOOSTING MENU

For those of you looking to rev up your metabolism, try these fat-burning recipes.

	BREAKFAST	LUNCH	DINNER	SNACK/DESSERT
Monday	Blueberry Pancakes with Blueberry Syrup (page 26)	Fajita Chicken Skewers (page 174) and salad	Slow-Cooker Pot Roast (page 206)	Ranch Dip (page 105) with veggie sticks (see page 102)
Tuesday	Chili Cheese Omelet (page 40)	California Muffuletta (page 84)	Manly Beer Chili (page 196)	Apple Pie Square (page 250)
Wednesday	Vegetarian Breakfast Sandwich (page 36)	Caesar Salad Wrap (page 72)	Chicken Tortilla Soup (page 182)	Orange Cream Ice Pop (page 254)
Thursday	Blueberry Pancakes with Blueberry Syrup (page 26)	Fajita Chicken Skewers (page 174) and salad	California Club Pizza (page 136)	Ranch Dip (page 105) with veggie sticks (see page 102)
Friday	Chili Cheese Omelet (page 40)	California Muffuletta (page 84)	Veggie-Packed Lasagna (page 156)	Trail Mix (page 109)
Saturday	Vegetarian Breakfast Sandwich (page 36)	Leftover Manly Beer Chili (page 196)	Fajita Chicken Skewers (page 174) and Black Bean Avocado Salad (page 192)	Orange Cream Ice Pop (page 254)
Sunday	Blueberry Pancakes with Blueberry Syrup (page 26)	Leftover Slow-Cooker Pot Roast (page 206)	Steak Fajitas (page 191)	Trail Mix (page 109)

NEW COOKS MENU

New cooks, this one is for you—easy recipes to help you increase your kitchen confidence.

	BREAKFAST	LUNCH	DINNER	SNACK/DESSERT
Monday	Vegetarian Breakfast Sandwich (page 36)	French Onion Grilled Panini (page 70)	Crispy Pan-Fried Pork Chops (page 204) and salad	Pineapple Mango Ginger Sorbet (page 252)
Tuesday	Homemade Pumpkin Spice Granola (page 34)	Chicken, Avocado, and Cheddar Quesadilla (page 94)	Weeknight Chicken Tacos (page 188) and Cilantro Rice (page190)	Guacamole Dip (page 104) with veggie sticks (see page 102)
Wednesday	"Jelly Doughnut" French Toast and Strawberry Sauce (page 30)	Leftover Weeknight Chicken Tacos (page 188)	My Mom's Salsa Rice and Chicken Bake (page 198)	Strawberry Banana Shake (page 236)
Thursday	Vegetarian Breakfast Sandwich (page 36)	French Onion Grilled Panini (page 70)	Sausage and Pepper Hoagie (page 78)	Dark Chocolate-Covered Fruit (page 251)
Friday	Homemade Pumpkin Spice Granola (page 34)	Chicken, Avocado, and Cheddar Quesadilla, (page 94)	Skinny Chicken Alfredo (page146)	Guacamole Dip (page 104) with veggie sticks (see page 102)
Saturday	"Jelly Doughnut" French Toast and Strawberry Sauce (page 30)	Leftover Salsa Rice and Chicken Bake (page 198)	Cheddar-Stuffed Turkey Burgers (page 166)	Pineapple Mango Ginger Sorbet (page 252)
Sunday	Homemade Pumpkin Spice Granola (page 34)	Leftover Skinny Chicken Alfredo (page 146)	Roast Beef Sandwich with Creamy Horseradish Spread (page 76)	Strawberry Banana Shake (page 236)

HAPPY KIDS MENU

Happy kids make for happy parents! Here's a menu that adults will love, but it's been created with picky kids in mind.

	BREAKFAST	LUNCH	DINNER	SNACK/DESSERT
Monday	Blueberry Pancakes with Blueberry Syrup (page 26)	Nutty Chicken Salad Sliders (page 74)	Skinny Sloppy Joes (page 82)	Homemade Applesauce (page 112)
Tuesday	Elvis-Inspired Peanut Butter Banana Waffles (page 28)	Mini Cheesy Pretzel Dogs (page 98) and Ranch Dip (page 105) with veggie sticks (see page 102)	Lemony Drumsticks (page 172) and Veggie Kebabs (page 179)	Strawberries and Cream Cookies (page 48)
Wednesday	Giant Breakfast Cookies (page 32)	Elvis-Inspired Grilled Peanut Butter Banana Panini (page 68)	Skinny Chicken Potpie (page 202)	Loaded Chocolate-Covered Bananas (page 256)
Thursday	Strawberry Scones with Lime Glaze (page 60)	Creamy Mac and Cheese (page 90)	Pizza Rolls (page 138) and Caesar salad	Chocolate Peanut Butter Dip with Fruit (page 114)
Friday	Blueberry Pancakes with Blueberry Syrup (page 26)	Mini Cheesy Pretzel Dogs (page 98) and Ranch Dip (page 105) with veggie sticks (see page 102)	Meat Lovers' Baked Ziti (page 148) and salad	Homemade Applesauce (page 112)
Saturday	Elvis-Inspired Peanut Butter Banana Waffles (page 28)	Nutty Chicken Salad Sliders (page 74)	Grilled Chicken Strips (page 176) and Amusement Park Corn on the Cob (page 178)	Strawberries and Cream Cookies (page 48)
Sunday	Strawberry Scones with Lime Glaze (page 60)	Leftover Creamy Mac and Cheese (page 90)	Cheddar-Stuffed Turkey Burgers (page 166) and Asparagus "Fries" (page 171)	Chocolate Peanut Butter Dip with Fruit (page 114)

TIME CRUNCH MENU

For those of you on the go, here are some fast meals you can make ahead of time so that you can eat healthy no matter how busy your schedule!

	BREAKFAST	LUNCH	DINNER	SNACK/DESSERT
Monday	Homemade Pumpkin Spice Granola (page 34)	Roast Beef Sandwich with Creamy Horseradish Spread (page 76)	Weeknight Chicken Tacos (page 188) with Cilantro Rice (page 190)	Dark Chocolate Chip Granola Bars (page 110)
Tuesday	Giant Breakfast Cookies (page 32)	Pesto Chicken Sandwich (page 86)	Sausage and Pepper Hoagie (page 78)	Chunky Blue Cheese Dip (page 108) with veggie sticks (see page 102)
Wednesday	Chocolate Chip Muffins (page 46)	Leftover Weeknight Chicken Tacos (page 188)	Chicken, Avocado, and Cheddar Quesadilla (page 94)	Chocolate, Banana, and Peanut Butter Blender "Ice Cream" (page 234)
Thursday	Homemade Pumpkin Spice Granola (page 34)	Roast Beef Sandwich with Creamy Horseradish Spread (page 76)	French Bread Pizza (page 142) and salad	Chunky Blue Cheese Dip (page 108) with veggie sticks (see page 102)
Friday	Giant Breakfast Cookies (page 32)	Pesto Chicken Sandwich (page 86)	Meat Lovers' Baked Ziti (page 148)	Chocolate, Banana, and Peanut Butter Blender "Ice Cream" (page 234)
Saturday	Chocolate Chip Muffins (page 46)	Leftover French Bread Pizza (page 142)	"Everything" Rubbed Steaks (page 168) and Veggie Kebabs (page 179)	Dark Chocolate Chip Granola Bars (page 110)
Sunday	Homemade Pumpkin Spice Granola (page 34)	Leftover Sausage and Pepper Hoagie (page 178)	Crispy Pan-Fried Pork Chops (page 204) and salad	Bananas Foster (page 232)

STAY-AT-HOME MENU

Stay-at-home parents have the luxury of cooking more time-consuming meals, but they should still be easy to toss together. Here are some of my favorites.

	BREAKFAST	LUNCH	DINNER	SNACK/DESSERT
Monday	Breakfast Scramble (page 42)	Skinny Sloppy Joes (page 82)	Chicken Fajita Enchiladas (page 186) and Black Bean Avocado Salad (page 192)	Rosemary Olive Oil Wheat Crackers (page 118)
Tuesday	Old-Fashioned Oatmeal with Topping Bar (page 24)	Leftover Chicken Fajita Enchiladas (page 186)	Creamy Mac and Cheese (page 90) and salad	Strawberry Shortcake Cupcakes (page 246)
Wednesday	Chili Cheese Omelet (page 40)	Grilled Chicken "Burger" (page 164)	Hawaiian Pizza (page 132)	Peach Sunrise Cobbler (page 244)
Thursday	Strawberry Scones with Lime Glaze (page 60)	Leftover Skinny Sloppy Joes (page 82)	Spaghetti Bolognese (page 150)	Rosemary Olive Oil Wheat Crackers (page 118)
Friday	Breakfast Scramble (page 42)	Leftover Spaghetti Bolognese (page 150)	Steak Fajitas (page 191)	Strawberry Shortcake Cupcakes (page 246)
Saturday	Old-Fashioned Oatmeal with Topping Bar (page 24)	Leftover Chicken Fajita Enchiladas (page 186)	BBQ Turkey Meat Loaf (page 203) and Twice-Baked Cheesy Potato Boats (page 92)	Peach Sunrise Cobbler (page 244)
Sunday	Strawberry Scones with Lime Glaze (page 60)	Grilled Chicken "Burger" (page 164)	Pork Chops in Red Wine BBQ Sauce (page 170) and Asparagus "Fries" (page 171)	Game-Day Nacho Dip (page 96)

VEGETARIAN MENU

Whether you're enjoying a meatless week or a meatless life, there are many options in this book to keep you satisfied!

	BREAKFAST	LUNCH	DINNER	SNACK/DESSERT
Monday	Old-Fashioned Oatmeal with Topping Bar (page 24)	California Muffuletta (page 84)	Pear, Rosemary, and Goat Cheese Pizza (page 134)	Loaded Chocolate-Covered Bananas (page 256)
Tuesday	Vegetarian Breakfast Sandwich (page 36)	Tomato Basil Mozzarella Panini (page 66)	Greek Pasta Salad (page 152)	BBQ-Flavored Potato Chips (page 113)
Wednesday	Homemade Pumpkin Spice Granola (page 34)	Leftover Greek Pasta Salad (page 152)	Veggie-Packed Lasagna (page 156; remove the sausage)	Tiramisu (page 240)
Thursday	Old-Fashioned Oatmeal with Topping Bar (page 24)	Caesar Salad Wrap (page 72; remove the chicken)	Margherita Pizza (page 126)	Loaded Chocolate-Covered Bananas (page 256)
Friday	Vegetarian Breakfast Sandwich (page 36)	Leftover Veggie-Packed Lasagna (page 156)	Overloaded Baked Potato (page 208; remove the chicken)	BBQ-Flavored Potato Chips (page 113)
Saturday	Homemade Pumpkin Spice Granola (page 34)	California Muffuletta (page 84)	Veggie Kebabs (page 179) and a tortilla	Tiramisu (page 240)
Sunday	Old-Fashioned Oatmeal with Topping Bar (page 24)	Tomato Basil Mozzarella Panini (page 66)	Vegetarian Stuffed Shells (page 154) and salad	Jalapeño Cheddar Scone (page 58)

Universal Conversion Chart

OVEN TEMPERATURE EQUIVALENTS

250°F = 120°C
275°F = 135°C
300°F = 150°C
325°F = 160°C
350°F = 180°C
375°F = 190°C
400°F = 200°C
425°F = 220°C
450°F = 230°C
475°F = 240°C
500°F = 260°C

MEASUREMENT EQUIVALENTS

Measurements should always be level unless directed otherwise.

⅛ teaspoon = 0.5 mL
¼ teaspoon = 1 mL
½ teaspoon = 2 mL
1 teaspoon = 5 mL
1 tablespoon = 3 teaspoons = ½ fluid ounce = 15 mL
2 tablespoons = ⅛ cup = 1 fluid ounce = 30 mL
4 tablespoons = ¼ cup = 2 fluid ounces = 60 mL
5⅓ tablespoons = ⅓ cup = 3 fluid ounces = 80 mL
8 tablespoons = ½ cup = 4 fluid ounces = 120 mL
10⅔ tablespoons = ⅔ cup = 5 fluid ounces = 160 mL
12 tablespoons = ¾ cup = 6 fluid ounces = 180 mL
16 tablespoons = 1 cup = 8 fluid ounces = 240 mL

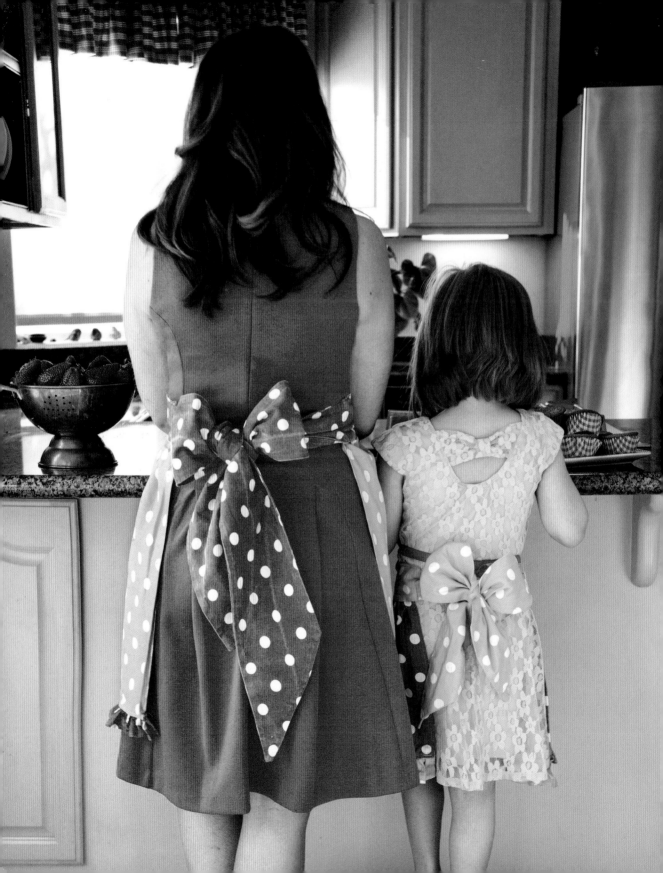

Acknowledgments

Many thanks . . .

To my partner and my love, Chris—thank you for supporting me in this wild life endeavor. Thank you for helping me test these recipes and for your honest opinion (even when I didn't want to hear it). To my little girl, Sophia—thank you for helping me stir, mix, and flip . . . and most of all, thank you for being such an amazing kid!

Kara, thank you for being my cheerleader for the last twenty-five-plus years. You are truly the best friend a girl could ever wish for.

Cassie Jones, I am so honored to have you as my editor—thank you for believing in and seeing my vision and for making me sound so eloquent. To my amazing agent, Celeste Fine—thank you for seeing this in me and encouraging me the entire way, and big props to your amazing assistant, Sarah, for always being available, calm, and knowledgeable. To my wonderful and talented photography and food styling team, Carl Kravats and Cindy Epstein and the Kitchen Princesses, Joni Wilhelm and Cherisse Holbert—thank you for making my work look so beautiful and making this process too fun to call "work."

I must also thank all my friends and family, whom I subjected to recipe testing when they thought they were just getting a free meal, and my wonderful extended family and in-laws for always being my cheerleaders. To my brave clients who helped me test this weight-loss plan and recipes—I adore you. This book is for you and all the longtime readers out there.

Thank you to my dear friend Kate for making cooking look so easy that I decided to pick up a spatula; to Laurie, who saved me during my first home-cooked Thanksgiving; to Brenda for letting me take over her kitchen; and to Marilinda for passing down amazing family recipes. To my team on *The Taste,* GO TEAM GREEN! I adore you, Sarah, Don, and Shehu! And thank you, Mom, for instilling in me the conviction that I have the power to teach myself anything I want to know, and that books and reading can open your mind. Your belief that anything is possible is the reason I embarked on this crazy food-filled journey. I miss you every day.

Last, to the kids out there being bullied because of their weight: much of my work came from wanting to prove my bullies wrong. Use their words to fuel you to do great things, and remember, you are beautiful at any weight! Beauty comes from within, and it is who you are, *not* what you look like. Beauty is found in your character, not on a scale!

Index

NOTE: Page references in *italics* indicate photographs.

Enchiladas, Chicken Fajita, 186–87, *187*

F

Fajita Chicken Skewers, 174, *175*

Fajitas, Steak, 191

French Toast

Almond-Crusted, 30

Bellini, 30

Eggnog, 30

"Jelly Doughnut," and Strawberry Sauce, 30, *31*

Fruit. *See* Berry(ies); *specific fruits*

G

Garlic

Bread, 56, 57

Bread Crackers, 118

Roasted Potatoes, 226

Rosemary Slow-Roasted Whole Chicken, 220, *221*

Grains. *See* Oats; Rice

Granola

Bars, Dark Chocolate Chip, 110, *111*

Homemade Pumpkin Spice, 34, 35

Gravy, Perfect Turkey or Chicken, 214, *215*

Greens. *See* Arugula; Lettuce; Spinach

Guacamole Dip, *103,* 104

H

Ham, Cherry-Glazed, 217

Herbs. *See also* Basil; Mint; Rosemary

Cilantro Rice, 190

Ranch Dip, *103,* 105

Horseradish Spread, Creamy, 76

Hot dogs

Mini Cheesy Pretzel Dogs, 98, 99

I

"Ice Cream," Blender

Almond Joy, 234

Chocolate, Banana, and Peanut Butter, 234, *235*

Freckled, 234

Nut-Free, 234

Ice Pops

Berries and Cream, 254

Orange Cream, 254, *255*

Tangerines and Cream, 254

L

Lasagna, Veggie-Packed, 156–58, *157*

Lemon Almond Biscotti, 50, *51*

Lemony Drumsticks, 172, *173*

Lettuce

Caesar Salad Wrap, 72, 73

Cheddar-Stuffed Turkey Burgers, 166, *167*

Roast Beef Sandwich with Creamy Horseradish Spread, 76, 77

Weeknight Chicken Tacos, 188, *189*

Lose Weight by Eating plan

buying food for, 14

drinking water, 9–10

eating all-natural food, 6–7

exercise, 8–9

goals for, 5

hitting the reset button, 10–11

ingredient notes, 14

logging your food, 8

meal planning, 7–8

measuring weight-loss success, 12

olive oil spray, 15

setting weight-loss goals, 11–12

skipping processed food, 6–7

Weekly Food Log, 16–17

Weight Loss Log, 13

M

Mango

Pineapple Ginger Sorbet, 252, 253

Skin-Firming Citrus Boost Water, 262, *263*